FIFTY SHADES OF FITNESS: GET FIT AT AGE FIFTY, AND BEYOND

FIFTY SHADES OF FITNESS: GET FIT AT AGE FIFTY, AND BEYOND

Supercharge Your Workouts

Dietrich Dejean
DTR Fitness, LLC
September 29, 2014

The information contained in this book is meant to maximize and supplement training for a sport or recreational activity competitive or noncompetitive.
Equivalent with multitudes and various types of training, the training methodologies discussed within this book do pose possible inherent risk. The author advises readers to take full responsibility for their safety, know their limits, and have a qualified coach or trainer supervise their programming. Before practicing the exercises or methods described in this book, be sure that your equipment is very well-maintained, and do not take risks far beyond your level of experience, aptitude, training, and convenience. As with many forms of exercise, please consult your physician prior to commencement of any challenging or strenuous activity.

ISBN: 1505638364
ISBN 13: 9781505638363

This book is dedicated to all my clients who helped me learn, grow, and succeed doing what I love. Helping you change your lives one day at a time has been my passion and my reward. Thank you!

Table of Contents

50 Shades of Fitness

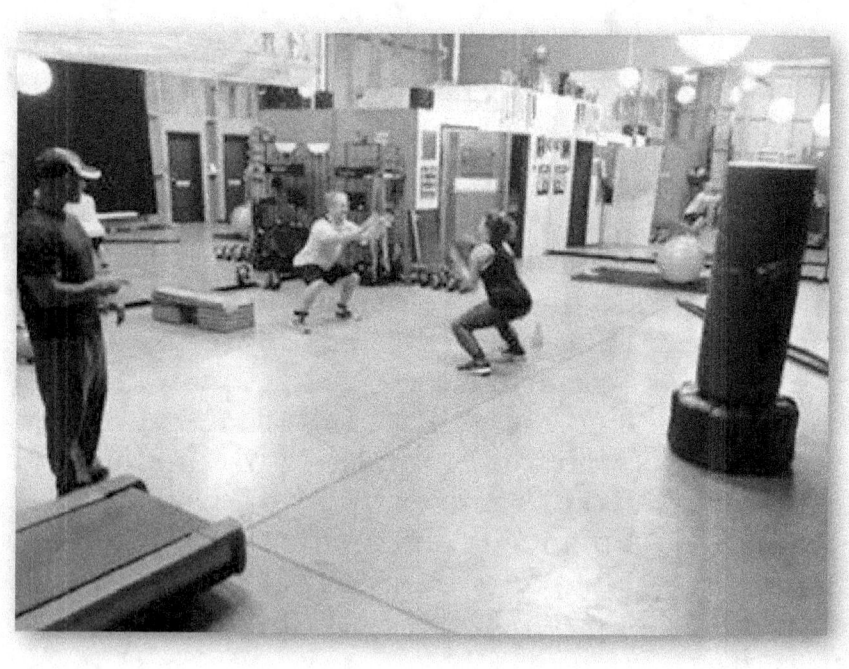

Introduction:
The Changing Lives Program

The realm of athletics is usually stereotyped as an area for younger people. Sports headlines are flooded with twenty-somethings making creative accomplishments and highlights in all different forms of competition. As soon as athletes such as tennis icon Serena Williams, soccer phenomenon David Beckham, or basketball superstar Lebron James reach their prime, the public considers retirement the next step. All the greats go through this. However, there is a set of competitors who buck the trend and refuse to deny their tennis shoes and racing bibs.

This is what masters athletes are: over-thirty-five adults who participate in any recreational sporting activity. There are plenty of champions and record holders in their forties, fifties, and sixties who compete at a high level and give evidence that age is just a number.

Masters athletics is a league of these over-thirty-five adults who defy the physiological breakdowns of the aging process. Events can be competitive or non-competitive, professional, semi-pro, or amateur. I've trained and coached athletes for many of these competitions, from track and field to weightlifting to ultra-marathoners.

This eBook will show you the methods and techniques to be a masters athlete, lose body-fat, defy the aging process, and restore vitality!

The main purpose of this exciting new fitness program is to change people's lives every single day. *Fifty Shades of Fitness* is a book to revolutionize the way mature adults approach fitness, increasing awareness and removing mental blocks to accomplish new active goals and promote long-term physical changes.

Active adults can accomplish their goals if they set forth with hard work, dedication, and knowledge of the mission at hand. Anyone, regardless of age or gender, can experience immediate extraordinary lifestyle changes by implementing proper exercise, resistance training, cardiovascular activity, flexibility, and nutrition. Active adults all across the world will have more awareness and confidence about their ability to maintain and sustain lifelong adherence to health and wellness. With the latest fitness trends and tools, you too can create maximum physical, mental, and spiritual well-being.

I have gathered tremendous research from over 12,500 documented training sessions and over eighteen years of experience in the personal training realm. I have trained hundreds of clients from teachers to parents to accomplished ultra-marathoners and senior athletes.

Imagine fitness regimens which consist of unconventional body weight exercises and exercise tools that focus on multi-joint motion, creativity, and functional movement patterns. Envision a program which helps an array of individuals, across the full spectrum of age and physical ability. This is what the Changing Lives Program is, and it will redefine how we view exercise and results. Now, let's get into the best shape of our lives.

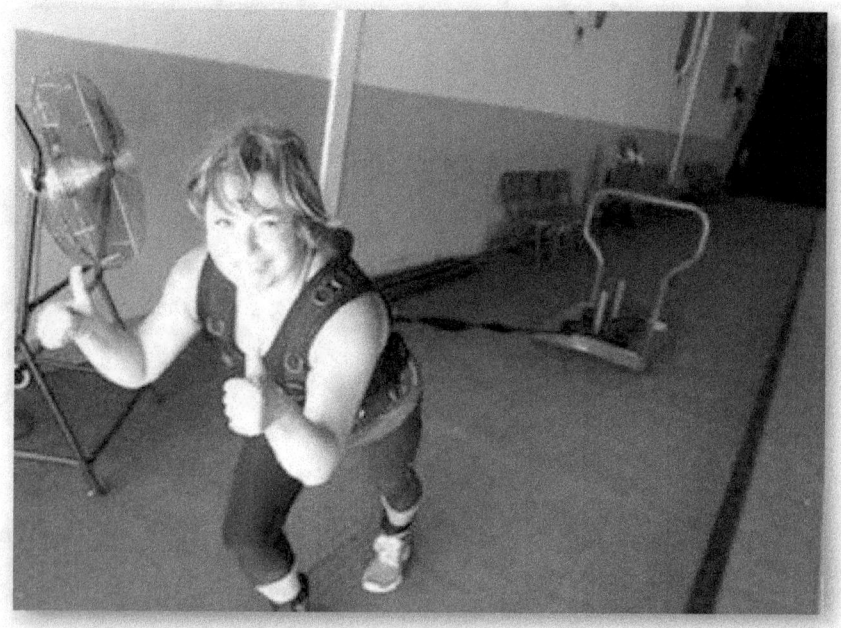

Natalia S. performing a sled pull with tubing on lower limb to perform conditioning and strength.

I

The Past

In April 2000, I suffered a major motorcycle accident and spent five days in an induced coma, two weeks on life support, four weeks in intensive care, and four months bedridden. I had hit a truck in a head-on collision, and one of my orthopedic surgeons even told me, "I don't know when you are going to walk again…" I had multiple compound fractures in my arm, thus could not write for a year. I had multiple severe fractures in my hip, thus could not walk for over a year. I used my doctors pessimism, and progressed from a wheelchair to a walker, from a walker to a cane, and finally from a cane to walking on my own at the end of 2001.

During my recovery, I learned many things about myself. Through adversity, I built my faith, determination, and willpower. I decided to compete in Olympic weightlifting competitions, build my own business in fitness, and go back to school to finish my undergraduate degree. I did not understand the importance of communication, problem-solving, writing, information retrieval, and collaboration in a professional setting until I finished my educational degree. Today, I'm an aspiring writer, an entrepreneur with a successful fitness operation, and a graduate from the University of Phoenix with a Bachelor of Science degree with honors. I've played semi-professional football and competed in powerlifting and bodybuilding.

These challenges are the backbone of the Changing Lives program. My experiences of failure to success are the true definition of what it takes to become a success in this health program. The goal is not to be just physically stronger, but to be stronger in all aspects of life. This includes strength of the mind, within personal relationships, and regarding career objectives, along with physiologically.

As I myself am over the age of thirty-five, with a history of competitive athletics, and still participate in recreational sports, I understand the necessity of establishing a program for older adults. Most of my clients over sixty know the importance of taking care of their bodies first.

Eat healthy, get rest. The older you get the more recovery time you need. When you're older, you have to be smarter with your body. The key element when aging gracefully is that you understand your body, and increase awareness. Unfortunately, this is an understanding many people do not have, especially after forty or fifty years of age. This is where the Changing Lives program and DTR Fitness takes effect.

Mission Statement

Changing Lives will continue to offer the most innovative, energetic, and fun approach to fitness. It is our mission to deliver this innovation through the most knowledgeable fitness professionals within the most unique fitness services in the world. DTR Fitness and the Changing Lives Program will constantly strive to be on the cutting edge of health and fitness, not merely following trends but setting them.

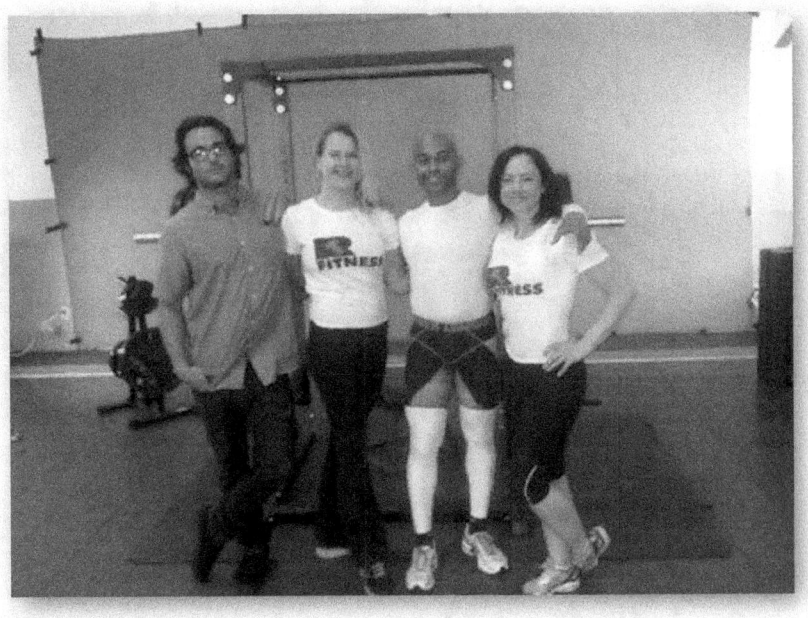

Business Philosophy:

The rise of obesity and health problems in children has become a growing epidemic. There are not enough programs or support systems for youths to participate in healthy activities. Changing Lives provides amenities, activities and an entertaining environment to engage families and children in their fitness education and participation.

1. Fitness specialists and experts hired by DTR Fitness and participating health facilities are college-educated only. As a college graduate myself, I believe the work ethic necessary for college is also imperative for understanding how to interact with clients and peers on a professional level. All fitness personnel executing this program must have a Health and Sciences degree and be CPR & AED certified. The fitness staff of each facility may be comprised of five to six members, including group fitness coaches, an expert yoga instructor, massage therapist, a strength and conditioning coach, and a Pilates instructor in an exclusive private studio. A potential client's first initial consultation

will include: a medical PAR Q (Physical Activity Readiness Questionnaire), health history questionnaire, goal assessment, body composition analysis, muscle balance assessment, and other vital information to help design an exercise and nutritional program.

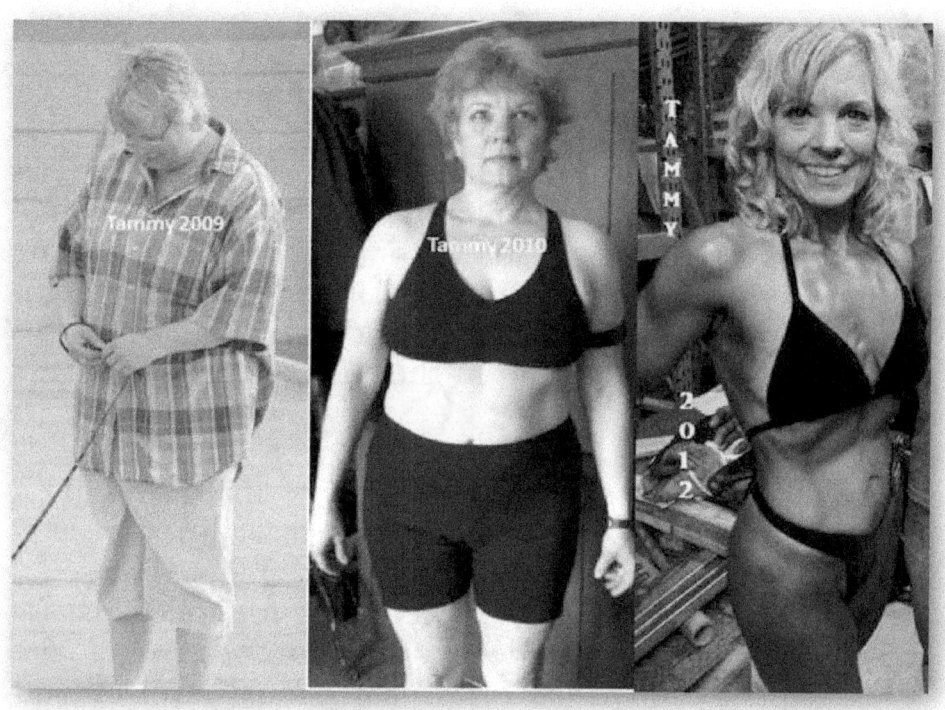

Personal trainer and nutrition expert Tammy H. White transforming, losing over seventy pounds of fat and becoming a fitness competitor after the age of fifty!

IMPORTANCE OF VISION

Vision is imperative in accomplishing goals and fulfilling objectives to facilitate a plan of action. Dealing with failure can inspire people achieve success. The most important instruction from Peter Senge's five disciplines in a human service organization is building a shared vision. However, one must develop the other aspects of disciplines to maintain a higher level of excellence (Lewis, **pp. 245-274,** 2007). Visualizing goals enables people to move forward. The vision for the Changing Lives Program is to use the latest fitness trends and tools to create maximum physical, mental, and spiritual well-being. The purpose is always changing lives.

Equipment such as TRX suspension training, kettlebells, sandbags, sleds, odd object equipment, yoga, mat Pilates, and body-weight exercises are key elements integrated in the Changing Lives Program. But to make the program work, qualified fitness professionals must have the "it factor." Trainers and fitness professionals who have the "it factor" possess passion, drive, ambition, high energy, persistence, dedication, charisma, charm, patience, and leadership qualities to help a client in a progressive and constructive manner for achieving goals. For instance, one of the mistakes I have made in the past is implementing the Changing Lives Program with knowledgeable trainers solely based on their credentials, certifications, and college degrees. This is not a fool-proof method to address successful facilitation of a unique program. Many clients who participated in a fitness program with a so-called "qualified trainer" did not get the results they wanted, mainly because their trainers did not possess certain attributes that a certification or degree cannot teach. Trainers failed to execute my personalized program because they did not possess passion, drive, ambition, high energy, persistence, dedication, charisma, charm, patience, and leadership qualities to help a client achieve goals. I created a Promotional DVD titled "How to Hire a Personal Trainer" to help professionals and clients understand the particulars and intangibles a qualified fitness professional must have to execute any training program. Possessing these necessary positive attributes is imperative to define success for the Changing Lives Program, and to excel in delivering proven results and optimal achievement of goals.

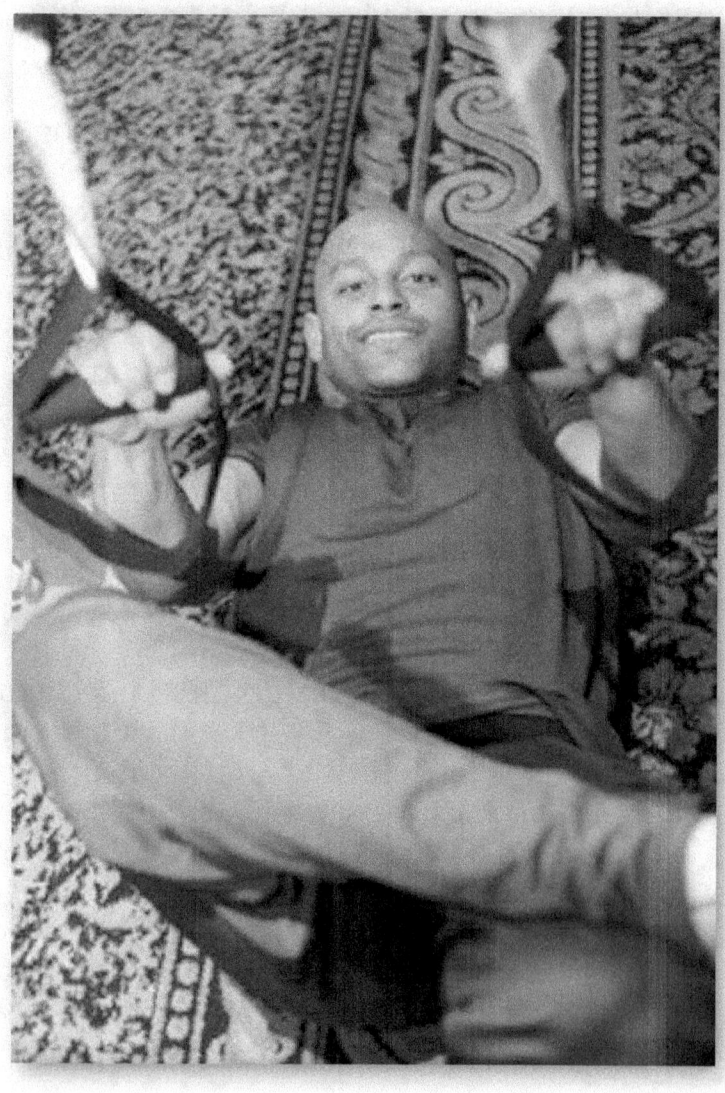

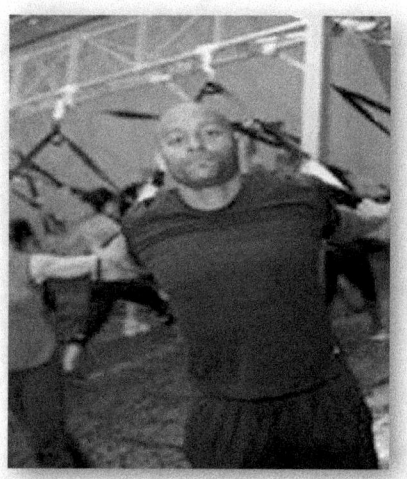

Dietrich Dejean performing TRX suspension training flexibility and strength drills

IV

Who is a Masters Athlete?

A masters athlete is classified as an over-thirty-five adult who participates in any recreational sporting activity. These sporting activities can be competitive and non-competitive, professional, semi-pro, or amateur. Active adults who fit this category all across the world have more awareness and confidence about their ability to maintain and sustain lifelong adherence to health and wellness.

Anyone can become a masters athlete. Many people with sedentary lifestyles, and a history of playing sports when they were younger, have gone on to become masters athletes. I've even worked with some masters athletes who had never had experience playing a team sport, but aspired to be a marathon runner or just to participate in cancer walks or fund-raising recreational activities. The Changing Lives Program helps all adults over thirty-five become more active and improve their abilities in a particular recreational activity.

Before DTR Fitness program:

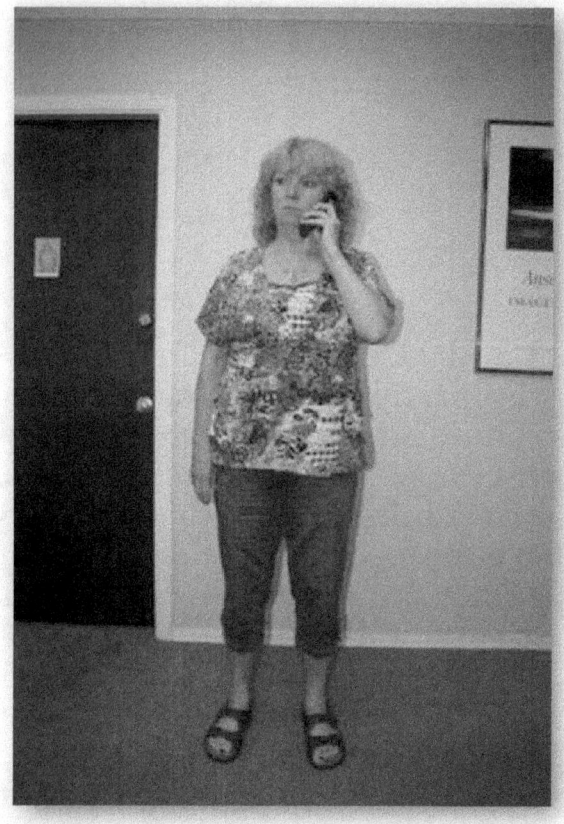

After DTR Fitness program (sixty pounds of fat loss at sixty-two years of age):

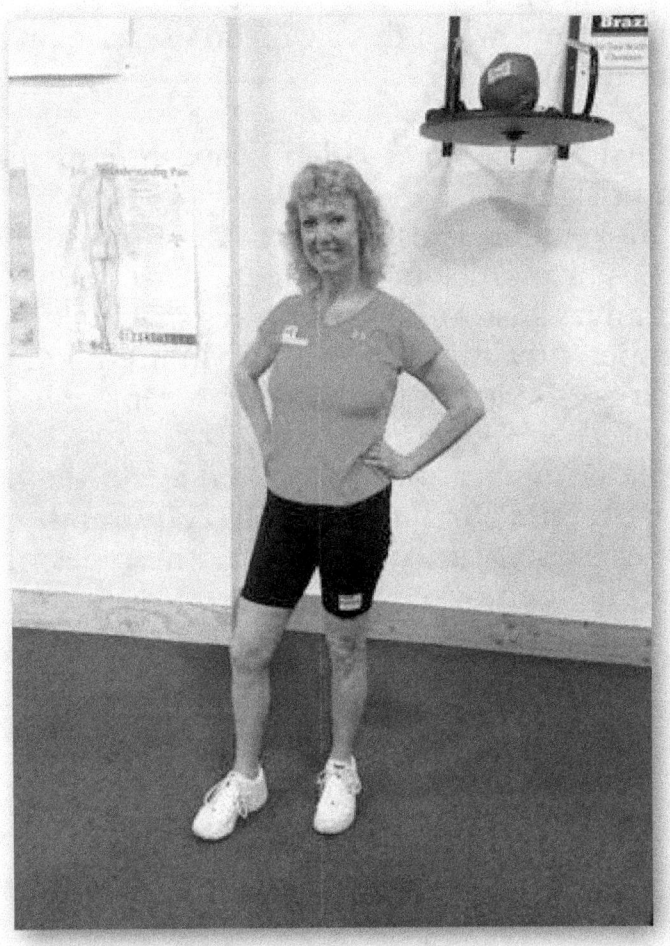

According to the National Strength and Conditioning Association (NSCA), the "fundamental principles of designing a resistance training program for an older person and a younger person are basically the same" (Baechle & Earle 2008). To design conditioning programs, the NSCA recommends a two-step process: evaluating the needs of the sport (or recreational activity) and conducting an assessment of the athlete (Baechle & Earle 2008).

Bearing this in mind, the Changing Lives Program requires these steps when designing an exercise program for a masters athlete:

- a health screening to identify existing medical issues and risk factors,
- a movement assessment to identify muscle imbalances or inefficient movement patterns,
- an injury history that identifies specific exercises for properly training a previously injured body part and exercises to avoid in order to prevent aggravating an injured area,
- a list of medications that could affect the body during exercise (Bryant & Green 2009), and
- an exercise history to indicate the types of exercise the client enjoys.

V

Scenarios

For the Changing Lives Program to work, one must understand key scenarios or developments that qualify a participant for the program. For instance, one candidate for the program – we'll call her Mary – is a single thirty-six-year-old mother of three. Mary has a difficult relationship with her children, does not communicate well with co-workers, exhibits poor fitness and health choices, and thus wants to improve her self-image. After a few months on the program, because of her accomplishments in improving her nutrition, sleep patterns, and increased physical activity, Mary is able to communicate better with family members, improve performance and interpersonal relations at work, and mend her relationship with her children.

Here is another scenario: a fifty-two-year-old participant who had a stroke a few years back has lost control of his left side of his body, is unable to employ normal functionality, and has terrible social relationships, causing him to become extremely introverted. After a few months on the program, this person not only improves his physical limitations, but also improves his social interaction with others. He even has friends and participates in normal day-to-day activities. All of these accomplishments have developed because of the Changing Lives Program.

Another participant named Gary is forty-three years of age and a quadriplegic who is confined to a wheelchair for the rest of his life. Because of his physical limitations, Gary is withdrawn and displays many signs of depression. Through extensive physical therapy and participation in the Changing Lives Program, Gary is able to become more functional and independent, which leads to improved social interaction with family and friends. Plus, Gary is able to acquire a position in the work force.

All these scenarios depict the extreme and dynamic properties that the Changing Lives Program offers. No other wellness program exudes the specific detail and precise plan of action to execute such amazing success for health clubs members.

Finally, Steve is a forty-six-year-old active adult and former professional skier. His main goal is to become a better competitive cyclist, without sacrificing his lean body mass. Steve is 5' 8" and 175 pounds, with 6% body-fat. How would a professional design and implement a program that accomplishes these goals? The science and methodology employed with the Changing Lives Program has been developed to do just that – achieve goals – with cases like Steve's and countless others.

VI

Key Elements

The key elements of the Changing Lives Program are conflict, personal reason to change, and a solution. The conflict aspect of the program identifies problems and barriers. A participant's personal reason to change focuses motivation and opportunities. And a solution maximizes a range of opportunities. All solutions that effectively change lives have three distinct phases: physical, mental, and spiritual.

Weightlifting is very popular for those between the ages of thirty-five and fifty-four. The National Strength and Conditioning Association suggests that strength training can improve strength and power for adults of all ages. Given the benefits of this type of exercise – preservation of muscle mass and higher metabolic function – strength training is my current "fountain of youth" strategy for anti-aging (Baechle & Earle, 2008).

"Resistance training may be the secret to keeping aging muscles young and aging adults functional and independent" (Kraemer, Fleck, & Deschenes 2012). Research comparing younger men to older men performing the same resistance training programs has found that the older men do experience strength gains and other benefits similar to those of the younger men (Candow et al. 2011, Hurley,

Hanson, & Sheaff 2011, McCrory et al. 2009, Baker et al. 2006, Harris et al. 2004). As they age, both women and men (although more often with women) suffer structural changes such as loss of bone mineral density and loss of muscle mass. Strength training helps to minimize these drastic changes and impedes the physiological changes during aging in men and women over the age of thirty-five. Myself and clients included in our program have shown tremendous results through the years and have never looked back. This is a life-changing phenomenon that people need to experience to enjoy a more fulfilling and active lifestyle. Functionality and vigor can be drastically restored with proper application of our programs.

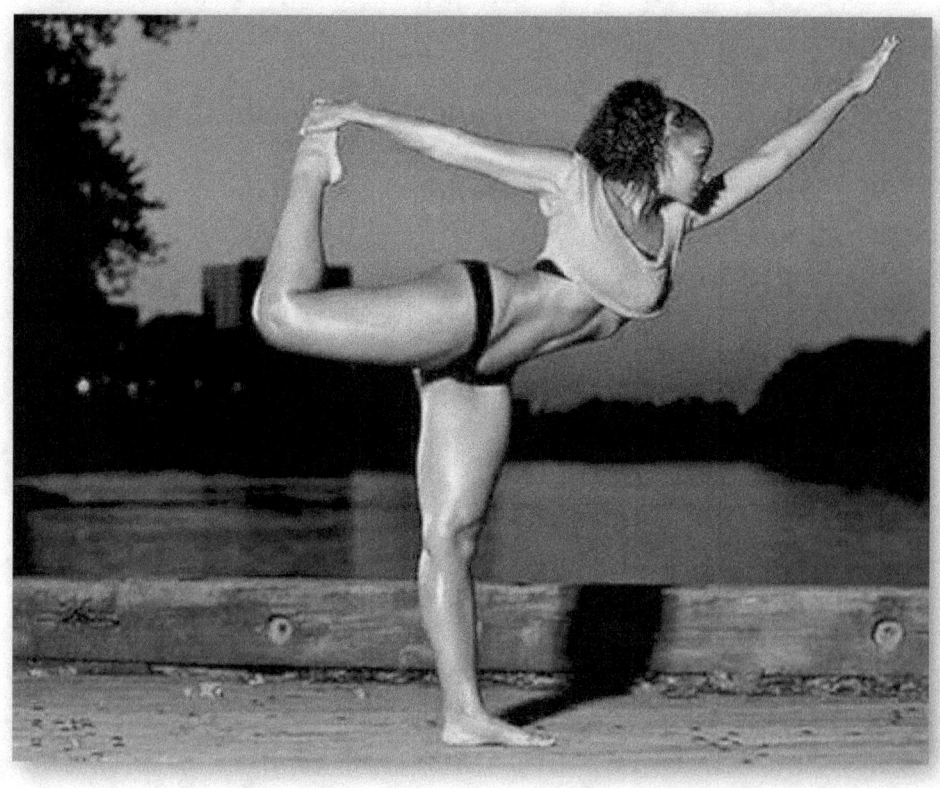

"Flexibility is important to ensure that aging muscle, fascia, and connective tissue remain pliable and elastic so that joints can articulate through their full ranges of motion" (McCall, 2013). The importance of flexibility is one of the reasons why yoga has become a hot trend coming into 2014. Dynamic flexibility and increasing the extensibility of the joints is crucial in the development of muscle tone and preventing injury as well. As we age, physiological demands display structural changes with the increase in inelastic collagen fibers. Combined with the lowered activity levels, the result is lack of flexibility and increase in the likelihood of muscle strains and other issues.

It is imperative to have a solid flexibility program for a masters athlete. Masters athletes have a number of disruptive and declining structural changes that are inevitable but can be alleviated with the proper implementation of a flexibility program. Flexibility ensures that aging muscles (especially after age thirty), connective tissue, and fascia remain elastic and pliable. This in turn helps the joints articulate full range of motion.

As the Changing Lives Program implements a unique flexibility program that is personalized for each participant, muscle extensibility and joint range of motion can not only be restored but can even be improved beyond the level it was at during the years of the client's youth.

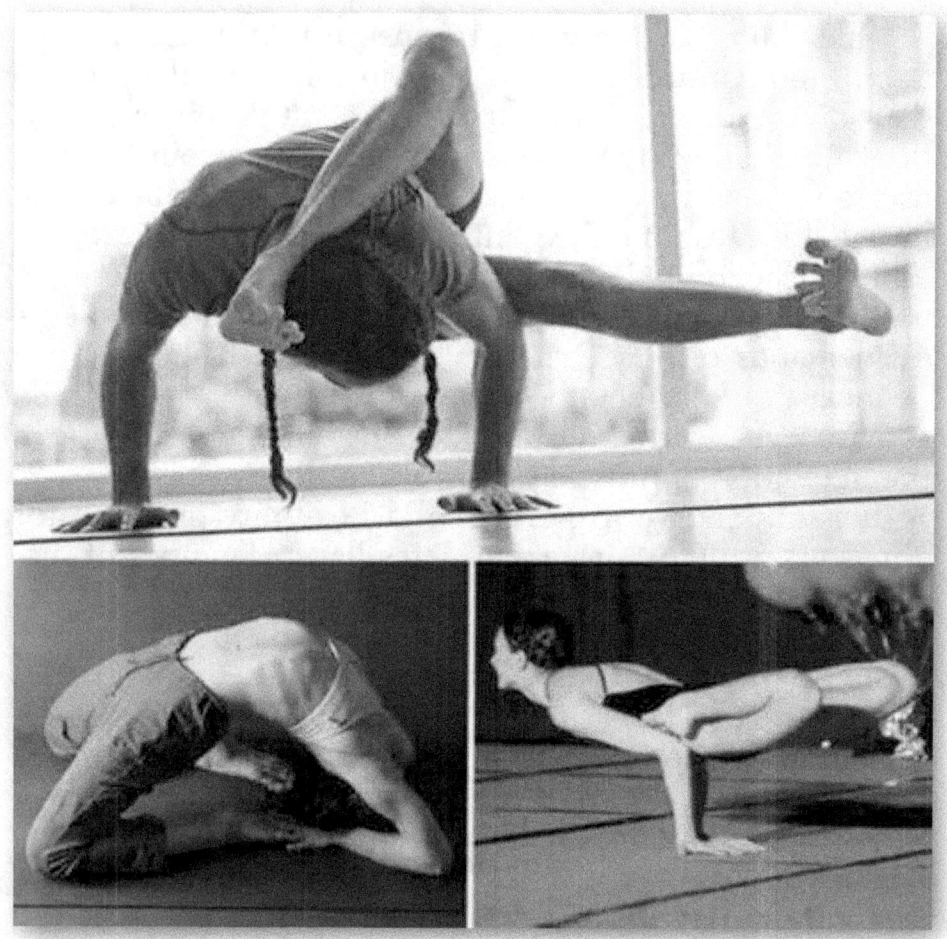

Advanced yoga moves to help aging muscles

Another key component for our Changing Lives Program is the importance of cardiorespiratory training, or aerobic programming. Certain physiological changes are inevitable during the aging process, such as the thickening of the heart's left ventricle and stiffness of vascular structures. Stroke volume declines and VO2 max (peak oxygen uptake) can decrease up to 10% per decade. The best antidote for all these physiological changes is implementing a properly structured program that helps slow down and reverse the normal aging process.

The Changing Lives Program implements many diverse applications of flexibility training, resistance training, and aerobic activity for qualified participants to achieve fast results. Coaches and professionals implementing the program should use isotonic, isometric, and isokinetic multi-joint compound closed-loop exercises as much as possible to maximize results for a masters athlete. Because of the ever-changing dynamics in recreational sports and the desire to have "fun" in fitness, the Changing Lives Program truly believes the necessity of implementing isotonic activities to transfer to real world functional ability and success.

FOAM ROLLING TO IMPROVE FLEXIBILITY

Foam rolling before and after an exercise activity or sport is a performance-enhancing application similar to the benefits of massage therapy and other similar self-myofascial release techniques. There are many types of rollers and sizes (I have even created one out of PVC piping and using a yoga mat to cover the pipe for a decent texture and surface), however the most popular one is the six-inch cylindrical shape made of foam that is usually two-to-three feet long.

Akin to Thai massage and deep soft tissue massage techniques, foam rolling reduces tightness and inhibitions in fibrous muscle tissues by applying physical loads of pressure. One has to be careful, because there are a multitude of techniques for proper application so he or she will not be predisposed to injury. Once muscles are released from tight inhibitions, muscles can retrieve better lengthening, elevate joint extensibility, and improve joint articulation. Applying these methods for just a few minutes per training session and on off days can considerably improve flexibility and strength. These physical improvements can also improve central nervous system response, speed, and muscle size or tone.

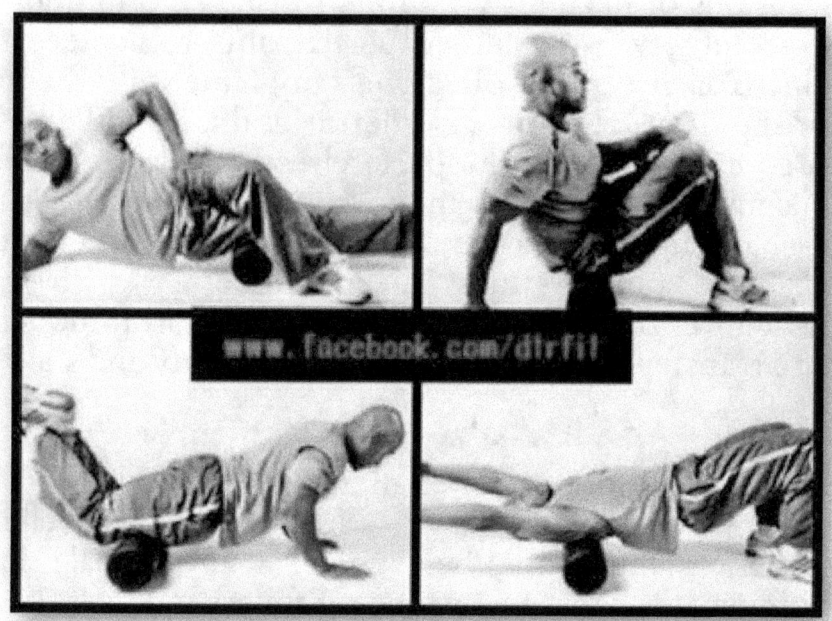

These are illustrations from an article I wrote in August 2011 for the Reno Gazette Journal to explain the benefits of foam rolling. Implementing proper foam rolling techniques can elevate a masters athlete's full potential.

Use the above illustration with this quick how-to guide for improving flexibility:

IT BAND (TOP LEFT)

- Place foam roller under left hip and assume Side Plank position.

- Balance on left elbow and right leg, and use leg to adjust intensity.
- Roll slowly from hip to knee, concentrating on sensitive areas.
- Perform on opposite leg.

Benefit: Reduces/prevents tightness and knee pain that results from overuse of the IT Band.

Variation: For maximum intensity, place feet together and off the ground or lift opposite leg.

GLUTES/PIRIFORMIS (TOP RIGHT)

- Sit with side of left glute on foam roller with opposite leg crossed over thigh.
- Balance on right hand and leg.
- Slowly roll back and forth over glute, concentrating on sensitive areas.
- Perform on opposite side.

Benefits: Reduces pressure on the sciatic nerve to improve nervous system control of lower body muscles and eliminate lower back pain.

Variation: Roll side to side over sensitive areas to release fascia from multiple directions.

QUADRICEPS (BOTTOM LEFT)

- Lie face down with foam roller under quads, balancing on elbows and maintaining a tight core.
- Roll slowly from knee to hip, concentrating on sensitive areas.

Benefits: Improves flexibility of these often over-developed muscles. Expands hip and knee mobility for improved jumping height and running technique.
Variation: For greater intensity, foam roll one leg at a time.

UPPER BACK (BOTTOM RIGHT)

- Lie on foam roller positioned at mid-back.
- Bridge hips toward ceiling and maintain a tight core.
- Roll slowly to upper back, concentrating on sensitive areas.

Benefits: Relieves upper back tension and pain, and improves back flexibility and shoulder mobility.
Variation: Roll sides of back for additional benefit.

For exercises that emphasize other parts of the body, either download my article online or contact me at DTRFitness.com.

Dietrich Dejean participating in program for cancer research (ACSM 2012 Summit):

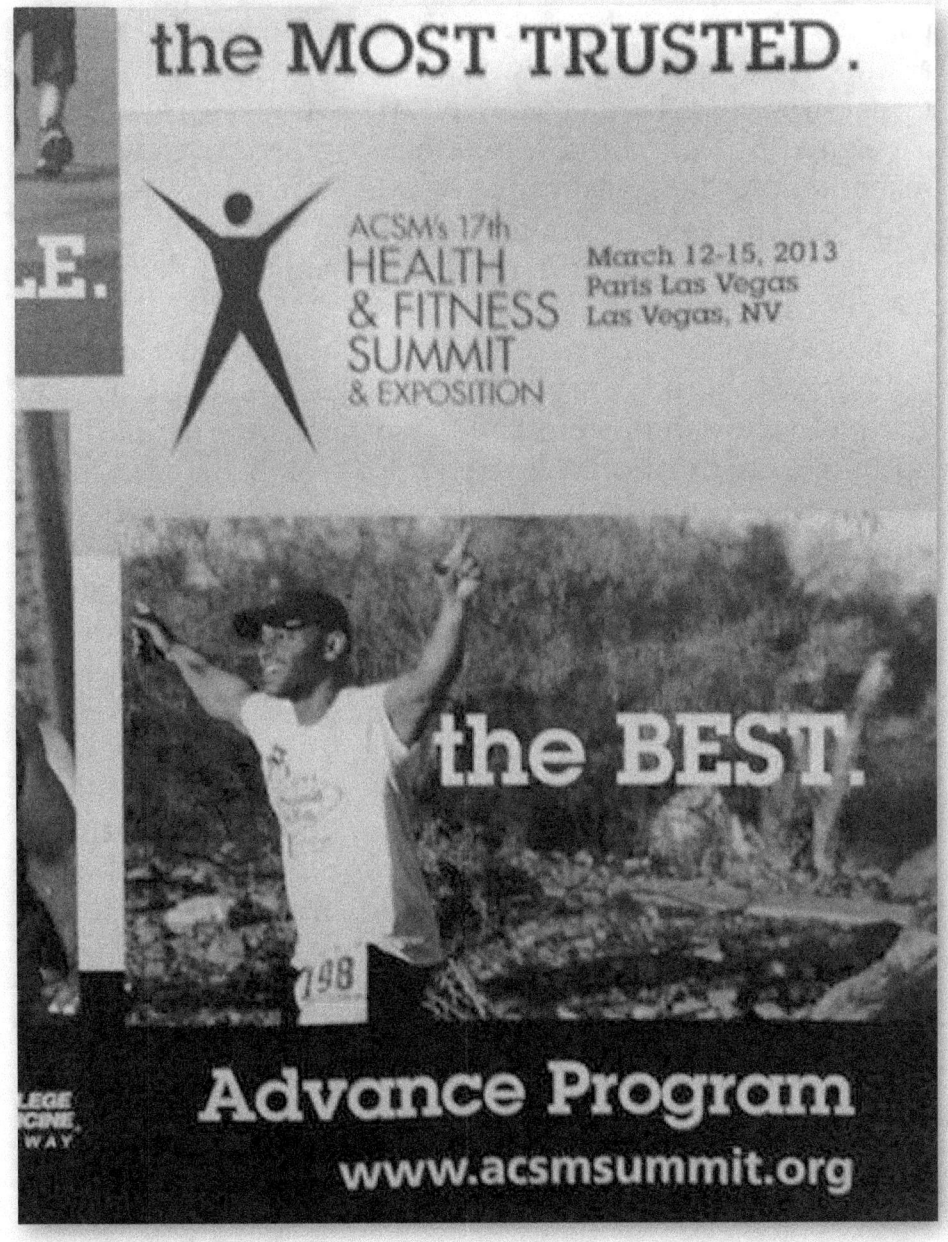

NUTRITION

Understanding the correct of macronutrient profile is important in determining optimal nutritional support for a participating masters athlete. From my experiences with adults over forty and fifty years of age especially, nutritional lifestyle accounts for over 70% of physical- and performance-based changes. Awareness must be elevated to teach people the significance of diet as it relates to losing body-fat, increasing vitality, reversing the aging process, raising metabolism, and most importantly, looking and feeling their best!

Recall the previous scenarios. How much fat and carbohydrates should Mary take in per day to accomplish her goal? How much protein and fat should Steve consume to optimize his hormonal levels and develop his lean body type, without sacrificing muscle mass to elevate cycling endurance and developing his aerobic energy system?

Micronutrients such as amino acids, vitamins, minerals, etc. are also crucial considerations. How can a professional recommend a supplement or vitamin without doing an assessment on a client? The Changing Lives Program requires participants to receive blood work to determine nutrient deficiencies and food allergen profiles. Blood work is vital to the development of the masters athlete. When we consume food as an energy source, our bodies chemically and organically break down the energy source in a multitude of ways. Every human being is different, and the process of gastrointestinal health and digestion is different in all adults as well. We are all special and different, and we must understand the complex systems and the beauty of how our bodies can physiologically absorb and expel nutrients. This includes not only the macronutrient level, but also micronutrient levels.

This is arguably the most important physical aspect, just as much as the recreational activity that needs to be addressed. If Steve cannot absorb a certain amount of protein or a type of protein, why should he consume it? What if he's taking 3000mg of Vitamin C, but his body is only absorbing 1400mg? Mary is taking 500mg of B-12. After seeing a specialist for blood work, it turns out her body can only absorb 300mg. Prior to seeing the specialist, Mary was overdosing on B-12 for a number of years. These are scenarios that occur with people on any normal given day.

Why should you sacrifice your time and body due to a lack of awareness? Why not fully optimize your ability to take in the correct amount of nutrients (either macro or micro) to maximize results? Seeing a blood specialist can determine all your deficiencies with macronutrients and micronutrients, such as Iron, Vitamin A, D, E, and other essential amino acids.

Our bodies need all twenty amino acids to make the complete proteins necessary for optimum muscle recovery. Eleven of these can be produced in your body, and nine must be consumed from foods. These are called essential amino acids, which derived from animal sources and soy-based foods. Most plant-based foods (vegetables, grains, legumes, etc.) are missing one or more essential amino acids. For vegans to get all the essential amino acids, they must consume different combinations of foods, like brown rice and lentils for example.

Muscle recovery is the process by which your muscles heal and adapt themselves to exercise. When you lift weights or perform heavy cycling or running, your muscles form microscopic tears from repetitive muscle contraction. Growth factor hormones get involved and develop satellite cells (containing protein and amino acids) to increase the enlargement of muscle fibers. These satellite cells travel to the site of damaged muscle cells and fuse them together, increasing the muscles' size. This process is like stitching a wound together. Some of the cells stay at the repair site and provide new nuclei for the recently healed muscle. This triggers muscle fibers to make more proteins, allowing the muscles to grow stronger and more resistant to future damage.

When you eat is just as important as what you eat when it comes to supplying the muscles with enough amino acids to grow. Post-workout, your body enters the anabolic phase, when you need to take in carbohydrates and proteins. Expert advice varies, but the rule of thumb I give my clients is to consume a four-to-one ratio of carbohydrates to protein.

The quantity of proteins you eat daily should depend on your body weight, gender, and health status. Registered dietitian Nancy Clark recommends that 0.5 to 0.7 grams of protein per pound of body weight if you're recreationally active. If you want to increase muscle mass or if you are an endurance athlete, consume between 0.5 to 0.9 grams of protein per pound for adequate amino acids to support growth. Remember Steve's case scenario and goals? To achieve Steve's cycling and lean body mass goals, a professional executing the Changing Lives Program has to implement a customized and tailored nutritional program design that combines a multitude of elements. If you weigh 150 pounds and are recreationally active, you should consume between seventy-five and 105 grams of protein per day. Consult a sports dietitian for your specific protein and other dietary needs (Clark, 2012).

The best choice you can make is to eat foods the way they appear in nature. You should choose fresh foods over canned or frozen foods, and natural, unrefined foods over more processed foods. For example, vegetables, potatoes, fruit, rice, and oatmeal are less processed and more nutrient-dense than crackers, enriched bread, pretzels, or bagels. When choosing your food, ask yourself this question: Did this food come out of the ground or off the plant this way?

Although the variety in your food choices is nearly infinite, there are staple foods that should make up the foundation of your diet. Variety will keep you enthusiastic about nutrition, but these are the foods you can't go wrong with, the foods you'll keep coming back to time after time.

The Terrific Twelve: The Twelve Best Foods You Should Eat All the Time

1. oatmeal and other whole grain cereals such as barley and rye (gluten-free substitutes if necessary)
2. 100% whole grain breads
3. yams and sweet potatoes
4. red potatoes and sweet white potatoes
5. carrots, turnips, and other root vegetables
6. leafy green vegetables
7. fresh fruit
8. coconut oil and olive oil
9. chicken and turkey breast
10. lean red meat
11. fish
12. egg whites – farm-raised and organic are preferable

Enjoy mixing and matching foods from the above list. Find new recipes online and have fun with them! But in order to keep your nutrition at its absolute best, also be sure to avoid the foods on the following list.

The Dirty Dozen: The Twelve Worst Fat-Storing Foods You Should Never Eat

1. ice cream
2. fried foods
3. doughnuts and pastries
4. candy, including processed milk chocolate
5. soda
6. fruit drinks and other sugar-sweetened beverages
7. chips
8. hormone-fed bacon or sausage
9. white bread
10. hot dogs or fast food burgers
11. cookies, cake, pie, and other sweets
12. sugary breakfast cereals

If you're in tears right now because I just took away all of your favorite foods, and you're wondering what the heck I've left you with, don't worry. I'm going to tell you exactly what new foods you can put in place of your old food choices. Although not all the alternative foods below are "A-grade," they are all improvements over their "low grade" counterparts.

Poor Choice	Improved Choice
whole milk	coconut milk, almond milk, non-fat or skim milk
white bread	100% whole grain bread, Ezekiel bread, or rye bread or lettuce wrap

ice cream	low-fat, nonfat, or sugar-free frozen yogurt, fruit sorbet, coconut ice cream, or frozen Greek yogurt
tuna in oil	tuna in water (or tuna with olive oil)
buttered popcorn	light microwave popcorn, or air-popped popcorn
regular crackers	100% whole grain crackers, rye crackers, or rice cakes
regular chips	baked chips or kettle-cooked chips
doughnuts	sugar-free, whole grain muffins or bagels, or butternut squash
fast food breakfasts	farm-raised, organic eggs
fast food, in general	protein bar or smoothie
regular cheese	low-fat or nonfat cheese
canned fruit in syrup	fresh fruit, or canned fruit in its own juice
sweets	fruit – low glycemic, such as berries, apricots, and apples
table sugar	Equal, Truvia, or Stevia
fried chicken	broiled skinless chicken breast

regular jelly/jam	all-fruit, no-sugar-added jelly
fruit drinks	100% fruit juice
soda	water, flavored with fruit or Crystal Lite
prime rib	round steak, lean sirloin, flank steak
regular butter	pure grass-fed butter
supermarket oils	coconut oil or extra virgin olive oil
regular cream cheese	low-fat or nonfat cream cheese
regular mayonnaise	low-fat or nonfat mayonnaise
French fries	baked potato or sweet potato
regular Jell-O	sugar-free Jell-O
sugary cereals	whole grain, low-sugar cereals
flavored, sweetened oatmeal	old-fashioned whole oats
regular ham, bacon, sausage, or hot dogs	lean ham, turkey sausage, chicken breast, or nitrate-free bacon
regular popsicles	sugar-free popsicles
gummi snacks	RAP protein gummies

MENTAL COACHING

Human psychology plays a significant role in an athlete's performance, as well as in the lives of adults who participate in a healthy lifestyle and/or recreational sport. Contrary to common belief, sport activities are 90% mental and 10% physical. Athletes should train the mind as much as the body. Mindset is the perfect part of the equation to deliver a success formula in any athletic undertaking. Mental imagery, focus, determination and visualization are key principles that need to be integrated to become a champion. Knowledge discerning mental coaching is paramount if one wishes to experience victory.

Air Force Rescue Athletes from California, Colorado, Texas, and New York travel to Bakersfield, CA for the RA (Rescue Athletes) Operation X (OpX) Air Force Battlefield Airman Prep Course. These athletes prepare for initial Battlefield Airman courses by training mental toughness, as well as management strategy and focus through rigorous physical circumstances. The overall focus of each OpX revolves around one critical fact: Battlefield Airman (BA) Assessment and Selection is 90% mental and 10% physical.

The time is now to acquire the proper mindset to succeed, and reinforce it with proper training. The muscles in your body are trainable, and so is your mental capacity. The mind has amazing capabilities; muscles have powerful capacities however have physiological limitations. Athletes cannot afford weaknesses in mental competence if they want to become a champion.

How many of you were championed athletes or tasted victory? What did it take mentally for you to achieve those goals? Who was coaching you to help you stay focused or implement proper strategy to make sure you were in the optimal space and time to succeed? If you have not yet been a champion in your life, would you like to know how you can be? How much do you think it would've made a difference to have improved mental coaching applied to your past or current capabilities? This is the base platform for our program. Sports psychology is imperative in the development of our physical well-being.

If you want to make the most of your athletic abilities, then you need to employ mental skills. Psychological factors are always manifested to affect athletic performance, no matter how much you or I prepare physically for a sport. Psychological factors, such as a lack of motivation and low confidence levels, are often the most challenging opponents for athletes. You play to win the game, but if you can't mentally capture it with focus, the right level of motivation, and utmost confidence, then your results will be disappointing.

Sometimes you hear athletes saying they are in the "zone." This is a key concept. Whether for team sports, powerlifting, running a 100-meter sprint, or doing a 5k cancer walk, being in the zone is like having the mental fortitude to telegraph how you're going to win, dominate, and become champion just by dictating superior mental skill (90%) with your physical aptitude (10%). The mindset is the cake, and the physical abilities are just the icing.

Mental imagery and visualization techniques are at the height of the proper forms of psychological training used by athletes. According to experts, the human mind cannot tell the difference between reality and imagination. Optimal performance can be achieved by simply drawing mental images and placing all energy and senses into your goal. You have the opportunity to manipulate your subconscious for your conscious brain to follow.

Mental coaching, more than anything else, is likely to help you get in the zone. Being in the zone gives an athlete the opportunity to meet the peak of his or her competencies.

The Changing Lives Program implements this concept at the forefront to achieve superior success for any masters athlete.

Fitness professionals executing the Changing Lives Program, and adults participating in the program, need to understand the importance of mental toughness. Experts define mental toughness as the ability to perform at your best in the most unpredictable and chaotic circumstance. Mentally tough athletes are passionate, optimistic, determined, and motivated. These qualities separate winners from losers and distinguish a leader from the rest of the pack in most sporting events.

Mental training can inhibit stress that might otherwise bother athletes. Athletes, like all people, are haunted by family and social demands. This might evolve as a major distraction along the course of the competition. Many benefits await masters athletes, with the implementation of successful mental training, other than acquiring athletic advantages. The goal of the Changing Lives Program is to develop the participant in all multidimensional aspects of life. The physical, mental, and spiritual capabilities of the masters athlete must all be raised in order to obtain higher levels of consistent performance and development.

While mental training comes in various forms and methods, they share common qualities for optimum athletic benefits. Commitment to goals, confidence in physical abilities, control of emotions regardless of distractions or underlying conditions, and the ability to stay focused and determined are all pivotal to achieving superior and consistent athletic performance.

The Changing Lives Program is not here to develop "one hit wonders." The goal is not a 400-yard drive off the tee in golf while still scoring double bogeys in each round.

Or being able to dunk a basketball but not shoot a free throw. What good is it to strive to finish a marathon but not resist those cream-filled doughnuts after a workout? The Changing Lives Program is developed to take adults to new heights that were thought to be unimaginable and incomprehensible. To boldly achieve results where they had never before. Such a feat requires discipline of both the mind and body.

This program warrants superior coaching and motivational strategies. Mental coaches aim to guide athletes in obtaining core mental skills. The qualified fitness professional knows the proper approach to help masters athletes overcome destructive mental barriers. Professionals possess the necessary skillset to help masters athletes set their achievable and highly desired goals. These concepts are imperative to jump start any mental training program and reveals that mental coaching plays a large role in excelling a masters athlete performance.

ENERGY SYSTEMS

Human physiology is simply incredible, capable of fascinating outcomes and physical endeavors. Our fitness programs for our clients vary depending on the energy system being used, goals of the client, and what is the most effective conditioning program for the client.

Two basic physiological concepts need to be considered when designing a conditioning program. Dr. Len Kravitz (who wrote over 200 peer reviewed research articles) states that the major source of energy used to perform activities must be recognized. There are three energy systems that our bodies utilize: two anaerobic energy systems (ATP-PC and lactic acid), and the oxidative energy system. The power capacity for the anaerobic energy systems is average to high while their capabilities to continue the work is moderate to low. On the contrary, the oxidative energy system has low power capabilities with a high capacity to carry on the physical activity. At any moment during training, it should be clear which of the three energy systems is being used. A trainer who is part of the Changing Lives Program will specify which energy system is being targeted (Kravitz, 1996).

ATP-PC (adenosine triphosphate and phosphocreatine) gives high power and low sustainability for work, with a time frame typically up to thirty seconds. The lactic acid energy system is more intermediate, with power time frames in the medium range and a work sustainability time frame of 30-120 seconds. Last but not least, the oxidative energy system exudes very low power output, and superior work capacity for optimal endurance.

The next step in the Changing Lives Program is developing a progressive overload system to develop whichever energy source is being targeted. Even if the overall goal is general fitness, the specificity of program design is essential to recognition. For instance, in general conditioning programs, perhaps all three energy systems will be involved, with emphasis determined by which system best meets the masters athlete's goals (such as programs like P90x and CrossFit). The Changing Lives Program is a unique method to develop masters athletes and optimize their results for whatever recreational activity they choose, which has become a new trend of awareness (Kravitz, 1996).

Cardiorespiratory endurance immediately affects the body's keen and acute adaptations by provoking numerous bodily changes in stroke volume, cell usage in carbohydrates and fats, aerobic respiration, blood flow within the muscles, and varying intensity in heart rates. Likewise, in resistance training the body's musculoskeletal system experiences alterations or physiological changes reflective of the tonnage or weights challenged.

Activity periods of time will also instantly affect the training effect from the proposed activity. Anaerobic training such as Olympic lifting incorporates repeated brief periods of high intensity exercise alternated with recovery periods in the training session. Continuous aerobic training embraces longer, prolonged periods of time of the activity at a lower magnitude.

Changing Lives conditioning programs vary in days per week (frequency). The degree of fitness of the masters athlete, as well as the level of training assist, defines the amount of days per week to take part in the physical activity. Ideally, The Changing Lives Program adheres to a frequency of three to five times per week over a period of three to four weeks with progressive changes and tapering to allow for maximum tenured programming for twelve weeks. This schedule will elicit adequate success for a purposeful training result. Experts have stated that maintaining a degree of physical fitness does not necessitate the frequency widely accepted to accomplish the training result.

The Changing Lives Program helps professionals with ease and acute facilitation. The challenge facing coaches and fitness professionals is how to best manipulate, overload progressively, and blend intensity, frequency, and duration with a variety of styles of activity, to help clients encompass their goals. Fortunately the Changing Lives Program is available to many fitness professional, which includes and not limited to high intensity interval training (H.I.I.T.) and interval-related circuit training (Kravitz, 1996).

VII

Training Examples & Methodology

CIRCUIT TRAINING

Circuit training was developed by G.T. Anderson and R.E. Morgan in 1953 at the University of Leeds in England (Sorani, 1966). Sorani implies that the term circuit referred to carefully selected exercises arranged in a consecutive manner, usually with nine to twelve stations comprising this circuit (with each activity enduring fifteen to thirty seconds with minimal or no rest). The Changing Lives Program usually uses variations of this model with five to twenty-five repetitions at each station of activity with about 30-40% intensity of one rep maximum with resistance. We may use handheld weights like dumbbells and kettlebells, sand bags, elastic resistance, calisthenics, mat Pilates, yoga, weightlifting, martial arts, and other combinations of unconventional types of equipment or careful creative multi-joint exercise to help a client.

Depending on the client, circuit training can be more anaerobic base or aerobic base. This is what makes the Changing Lives Program second to none, because it recognizes the needs of the client first and then adapts and configures a training program to fit those needs.

Circuit 1

1. Pushups (might be varied depending on client level of fitness and ability – from one arm pushup to pushups using a stability ball)
2. Squats (might be varied to a Ball Squat with one leg, or an overhead squat with a dowel or Barbell, depending on client goals, muscle imbalances, and compensation points)
3. 2-3 minute aerobic activity such as jogging rowing walking uphill or with backpack, or cycling
4. Row pull (could use Barbell, TRX suspension training, dumbbell, kettlebell, or resistance band
5. Handstand
6. 2-3 minute aerobic activity
7. Overhead weighted press
8. Pull-ups
9. 2-3 minute aerobic activity
10. TRX bicep curl
11. TRX tricep extension
12. 2-3 minute aerobic activity (KB Swings and jump rope are great examples)

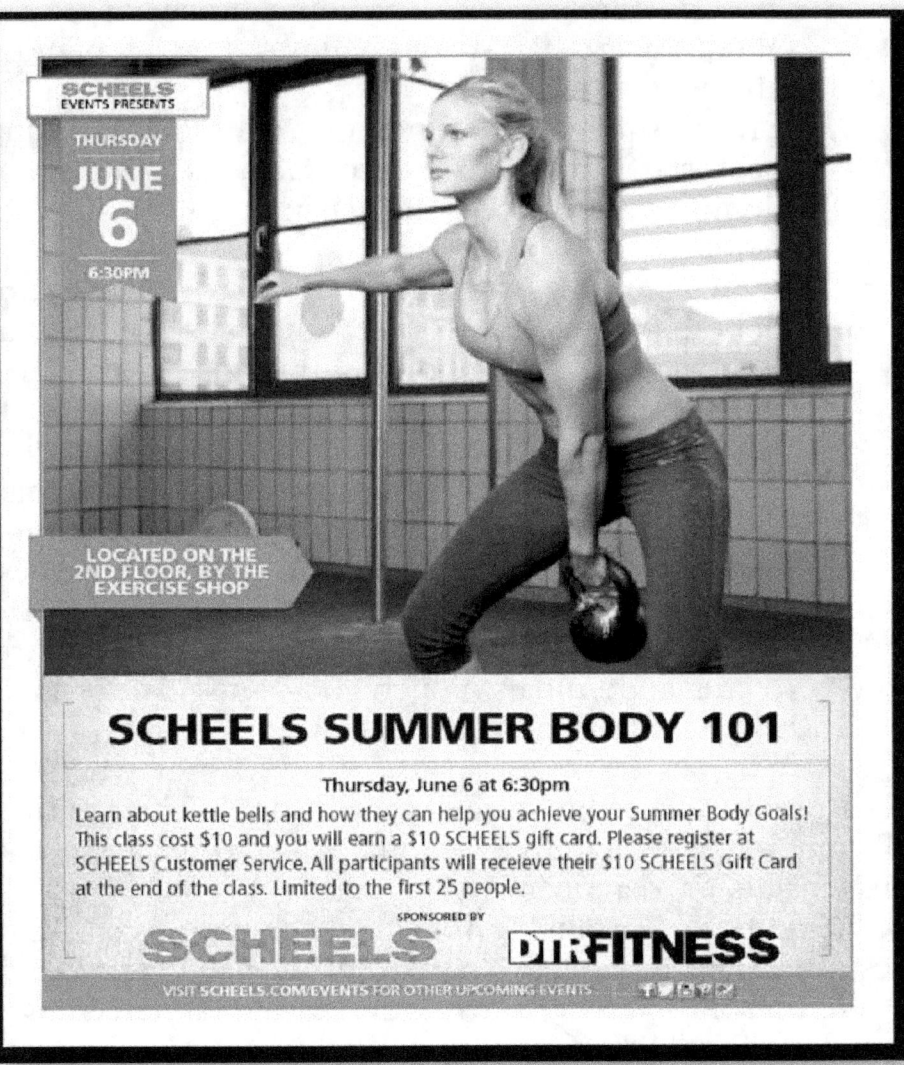

Circuit 2 (shown with the muscle groups involved)

1. Barbell overhead jerks (focusing on deltoid, trapezius, pectorals-clavicular, coracobrachialis, rectus abdominals, hamstrings, glutes, gastrocnemius, and soleus)
2. Front squats (focusing on deltoid, trapezius, pectorals-clavicular, coracobrachialis, rectus abdominals, quadriceps, hamstrings, glutes, gastrocnemius, and soleus)
3. Renegade row with pushup (pectorals, anterior deltoid, triceps, coracobrachialis, subscapularis, latissimus dorsi, rhomboids, infraspinatus, and teres minor)
4. Lunge with bicep curl to rotation (biceps brachii, brachialis, brachioradialis, quadriceps, hamstrings, glutes, gastrocnemius, soleus, core musculature, rectus abdominals, internal, and external obliques)
5. Box jump with one leg (quadriceps, hamstrings, glutes, gastrocnemius, soleus, core musculature, rectus abdominals, upper body musculature, pectorals, deltoids, biceps, and triceps brachii)

Note: the preceding circuit may be done with a variety of equipment, such as free weights, elastic resistance, strap suspension, or a sandbag.

Benefits of circuit training are numerous. Circuit resistance-training has displayed elevated muscular strength from 7% to 32% while decreasing fat percentages from 2.9% to 0.8% (Gettman & Pollock, 1981). Gettman and Pollock's review of the literature also showed an increase of fat-free weight (1 to 3.2 kg) with no subsequent change in body weight. Kilocalorie expenditure has been estimated to be approximately 5-6 kcal per minute for women and 8-9 kcal per minute for men (Hempel & Wells, 1985; Wilmore, Parr, & Ward, 1978). Furthermore, proper implementation of circuit resistance-training does not elevate resting blood pressure or heart rate, and may in fact lower resting diastolic blood pressure in borderline hypertensives (Harris & Holly, 1987). The psychological benefits as well are plentiful, with positive changes in mood, anxiety, depression, and hostility (Norvell & Belles, 1993).

INTERVAL TRAINING

Interval training has taken many strides and developments in the last half century. From popular exercise tapes and videos to Tabata training and CrossFit programs, high intensity interval training and normal interval training programs are a trend that are here to stay, especially in the "I don't have a lot of time to waste in the gym" mentality of our society. Let's face it, people are more impatient now than ever before.

Interval training varies the intensity within the training session by positioning a work period of a higher intensity with a rest period of lower intensity throughout the workout. This method of training is credited to Dr. Woldemer Gerschler of Germany who pioneered it around 1930 (Stone & Kroll, 1986). The work interval with high intensity effort directs which energy systems are being targeted.

In theory, a big advantage of interval training for our masters athletes is to help overload the heart briefly, beyond what could be accomplished during a single work period at similar intensity levels. In resistance training, muscles respond to the load of weight and the total reps performed, whereas in interval training, the resistance the heart overcomes is related to greater ventricular filling from enhanced venous return. This leads to higher contractility, which therefore encourages more complete emptying. Many busy people who do not have enough time in their hectic schedules welcome the alternating work and recovery periods in interval training to achieve more cardiovascular training.

General Guidelines for Designing Interval Training Fitness Programs

Energy System	Time Cycles	Number of Intervals	Sets	Recovery Ratio	Recovery Time	Type of Recovery
ATP-PC	0-30 sec.	8 – 10	1 – 5	1/3	0-90 sec.	passive
Lactic Acid	30-60 sec.	1 – 5	2 – 3	1/3	90-180 sec.	active or passive
Lactic Acid	60-120 sec.	1 – 5	2 – 3	1/2	120-240 sec.	active or passive
Oxidative	2-3 min.	4 – 6	1 – 2	1/2	4-6 min.	active or passive
Oxidative	3-5 min.	3 – 6	1 – 2	1/1	3-5 min.	active or passive

Modified from (Kravitz, 1996),(Mathews & Fox, 1976).

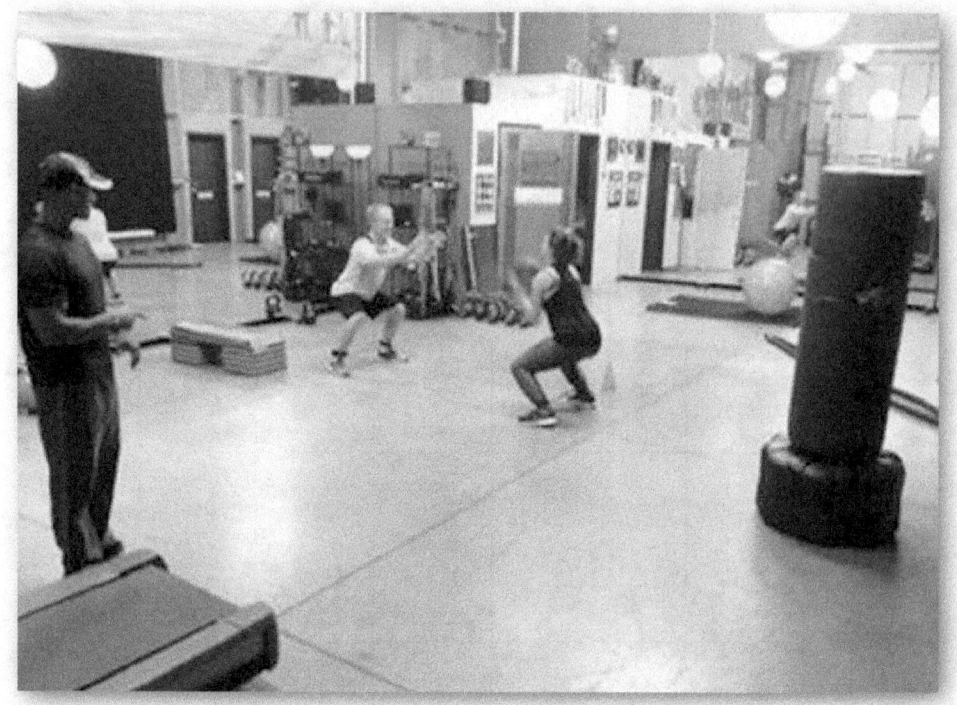

DTR Fitness clients and trainers participating
in an interval training program.

Interval training is not better than continuous training to maximize VO2. There are plenty of debates and
strong arguments to suggest otherwise, but according to
Dr. Kravitz, there is no research data that conclusively
supports one form of training to be superior to the other. I truly believe in finding a balance between various
methods to apply to a masters athlete participating in the
Changing Lives Program to achieve the best maximum results. Interval training helps with usage of carbohydrate
and fats, stimulates both fast and slow twitch muscle fibers,
improves anaerobic and aerobic power, improves weight
management, enhances physical ability, elevates sports
performance, reduces injury based on workout intensity

and overloading, and last but not least, produces greater work output in a shorter period of time!

Interval training and circuit training systems are magnificent for elevating physical fitness and exercise performance. These techniques can bring variety and fun to masters athletes, or any participating client in the Changing Lives Program. Professionals are encouraged to combine the science bestowed above with your own unique creativity and organization of new interval and circuit training programs for your classes and clients. We have adopted these findings and research to implement a new trend to elevate and enhance physical and mental aptitude in today's masters athlete.

UPPER-LOWER BODY INTERVAL CIRCUIT EXERCISE SAMPLES USED IN CHANGING LIVES PROGRAM

When alternating exercises with step training, the client may wrap the elastic resistance band around one hand or the waist. Doing so erases the participant's need to bend to pick up and put down the elastic resistance. This saves monumental amounts of time in our busy complex world.

Shoulder Press with Lunge

Put one foot on the step and one foot on the elastic band in a lunge position. Hold the elastic band next to the shoulders. Extend the arms upward as you lunge downward in the lunge. Return to starting position. Cycle alternating single and double arm shoulder presses.

Squat with Triceps Extension

With the arms held behind the head, descend into a squat while extending the arms outward. As the legs extend from the squat slowly bring the arms to the beginning position. Cycle doing sets of single alternating and double arm triceps extensions.

Lunge with Arm Extensions

Stand with elastic band under foot on step, with rear leg two and a half to three and a half feet back. Concentrate on lowering down to a ninety-degree-angle lunge with the front leg as the arms move back, past the side of the torso. Keep the palms facing backward during the action. Return to starting position. Do fifteen to twenty repetitions and switch to other leg.

Squat with Bicep Curl

Squat with the legs about shoulder-width apart, making sure the knees travel over the ankles. (Concentrates on posterior muscle recruitment as opposed to the knees and toes.) Curl the arms at the elbow as you squat down. Return to starting position. Cycle doing sets of single alternating and double arm biceps curls.

Squat with Row

Standing with legs shoulder-width apart and arms extended in front of the torso, cross the handles of the elastic band. While squatting down, pull the wrists towards torso, lifting the elbows vertically. Lower slowly to the starting position. Cycle alternating sets of single and double arm rows.

Side Lunge with Single Arm Crossing Over

Stand with one foot on step, on top of the elastic band, holding handle slightly above the knee. Keeping a slight bend at the elbow, bring the arm across the midline of the body. Hand is facing the direction of movement. As arm begins crossing midline of body, perform a lunge (with leg on step) in same direction of arm. Do fifteen to twenty-five repetitions with both arms.

ECCENTRIC RESISTANCE TRAINING

At the ACSM summit and exposition (2010 and 2012), I was able to discuss with Dr. Len Kravitz and proposed what method of resistance training is optimal to increase strength and power. The topic of eccentric training was intriguing to me, and he was presenting a course on the subject. I proceeded to probe Dr. Kravitz one-on-one regarding his research findings.

An eccentric muscle action is designed to protect our joint structures from damage by braking, or opposing force energy, in response to shortening actions known as concentric movement. In an eccentric action, the muscle elongates when tension caused by opposing force (such as a Barbell or Kettlebell load) is greater than the force yielded by the muscle.

With eccentric training, the body continues to burn calories for many hours after the exercise bout. H.I.I.T training and other traditional forms of resistance training show very high yields of Excess Post-exercise Oxygen Consumption (EPOC). The greatest EPOCs (afterburn after workout) ever recorded by studies and research were by H.I.I.T. and resistance strength training, but eccentric training knocks them both out of the park! This has been scientifically proven in the last few years.

Since the goal of the Changing Lives Program is to achieve a maximum rate of body fat loss, EPOC is targeted and maximized as much as possible, substantially elevating the total number of calories burnt that day. This groundbreaking discovery is only a few years old, and is the design and implementation of exercise programming, effectiveness, and research. Scientific studies, including my own data of empirical evidence, displays that participating clients from a 2007 to 2014 study elevated calorie burn more so than circuit or high intensity interval training. Interval training is still a segment of the Changing Lives Program, however it is not the focus or foundation of the program. There are many elements of the Changing Lives Program, and one needs to understand the importance of each element, and what each method prescribes to a masters athlete.

Most of the classical muscle load studies in exercise physiology have focused on isometric (same length) and isotonic (shortening) contractions. One of the first research observations on eccentric muscle actions took place in 1882, when Adolf Fick discovered that a contracting muscle under stretch could produce a greater force than a shortening muscle contraction (Lindstedt, LaStayo & Reich 2001). Approximately fifty years later, A.V. Hill (who became a Nobel laureate) discovered that the human body had a lower energy demand during an eccentric muscle action than during a concentric muscle action (Lindstedt, LaStayo & Reich 2001). Popular programs such as CrossFit and Vinsanity are effective and successful, but not as effective as implementing a creative and structured eccentric program. This is where the Changing Lives Program has a huge advantage and will revolutionize the fitness industry.

One of the great advantages of eccentric training, is the possibility of training every day without any ill effects and maintaining low risk with injury. With a qualified professional, the athlete can burn more calories and heat energy, especially after workouts, than ever imagined.

Lindstedt, LaStayo, and Reich note that in 1953 researcher Erling Asmussen introduced eccentric exercise as "excentric," with "ex" meaning "away from" and "centric" referring to the "center." When weight exceeds the force developed by the muscle, as in an eccentric muscle action, the exercise is referred to as negative work because the muscle is absorbing energy in this loaded motion. Overload principles and methods in resistance training have benefited from this for decades. Trainees, athletes, and coaches have been using these methods for years and until now have never fully understood the physiological empirical evidence that supports the magnitude of eccentric training (Jackson, Bubbico, & Kravitz, 2010).

PHYSIOLOGICAL MECHANISMS OF CONCENTRIC AND ECCENTRIC ACTIONS

Muscle is tension-producing tissue comprising of small contractile units referred to as sarcomeres (see Figure 1). Each sarcomere contains thick (myosin) and thin (actin) myofilaments (muscle filaments or proteins), which overlap to allow for the formation of a cross-bridge bond. The cross-bridge (or sliding-filament) theory of muscle contraction states that the shortening of a muscle occurs as the myosin cross-bridges cyclically attach to actin and draw the actin across the myosin, thereby creating force and shortening (Herzog et al. 2008).

Herzog and colleagues state that each of the cross-bridge attachment and detachment cycles is powered by the splitting of one molecule of adenosine triphosphate (ATP). This shortening contraction cycle is referred to as a concentric action (or contraction). Examples of activities in which concentric muscle actions occur include walking on level ground, kicking a ball, and picking up a weight.

An eccentric muscle contraction, on the other hand, is the stretching of a muscle in response to an opposing force on that muscle, when the opposing force (weight being lifted) is greater than the muscle's current force production. Herzog and colleagues (2008) propose that when the myofilaments of a muscle fiber are stretched while contracting (i.e. doing an eccentric contraction), there may be a decreased rate of cross-bridge detachments (thus an increased percentage of cross-bridges remain attached), leading to greater force production on the eccentric bout. In addition, Herzog et al. state that there is an increase in the stiffness of the titin protein (largest protein discovered in the human body) during an eccentric contraction. Titin adds a passive force enhancement, a tautness, to the muscle's force production while being lengthened, or under load (Jackson, Bubbico, & Kravitz, 2010).

Examples of activities in which eccentric muscle contractions occur include walking down a hill, and resisting the force of gravity while lowering a weight or object. Eccentric actions place a stretch on sarcomeres to the point where the myofilaments may experience sarcomere strain, or damage referred to as exercise-induced, delayed-onset muscle soreness (DOMS).

Moreover, series of events leading to DOMS from eccentric exercise displays many variables, adaptations, and physiological responses. All types of muscle contractions, especially in untrained individuals, can cause DOMS, but it is especially noticed after a bout of eccentric exercise. DOMS is typically characterized as the muscle soreness and swelling that become evident eight to ten hours after exercise and peak twenty-four to forty-eight hours after the activity (Balnave & Thompson 1993).

There are various theories explicating the multifaceted causes of DOMS. One hypothesis is a widely known cellular theory of DOMS that focuses on the irreversible strain placed on sarcomeres during an eccentric contraction, resulting in disruption of components within the sarcomeres, specifically the Z line and A band (McHugh et al. 1999). Another hypothesis is the connective-tissue theory, which emphasizes the disruption of non-contractile elements (i.e. connective tissue) in sarcomeres (such as the sarcoplasmic reticulum) and of connective tissue surrounding muscle proteins, or sarcolemma (McHugh et al. 1999).

A newer theory spotlights disruption of the excitation-contraction (E-C) coupling mechanism of the myosin cross-bridges attaching to actin proteins as an additional contributor to DOMS (Proske & Allen 2005). Lamb (2009) explains that the sarcoplasmic reticulum is "stretched" significantly during an eccentric contraction, resulting in an uncontrolled release of calcium ions (from the sarcoplasmic reticulum) into the cell fluid which is referred to as sarcoplasm. According to Lamb, this event results in a disruption of the voltage-regulating sensors in the sarcomeres (which regulate neural input in the muscle) and also contributes to DOMS occurring from the eccentric exercise (Lamb 2009).

With various theories about what causes DOMS, we are just beginning a saga of much to be learned through research.

REPEATED-BOUT EFFECT OF ECCENTRIC TRAINING

One area of research that has much promise in relation to DOMS and eccentric exercise is the repeated-bout effect (RBE). One of the only ways, it seems, to prevent or lessen

DOMS from eccentric exercise, or to hasten recovery from it, is to eccentrically stimulate the muscles about one week (or more) prior to the eccentric training bout (Pettitt et al. 2005). The reduced DOMS response to eccentric resistance, after the prior eccentric exposure, is referred to as the RBE.

Several studies have shown that performing a bout of exercise leading to DOMS and then repeating the eccentric bout of exercise several days (up to six months) later results in significantly lower levels of DOMS, reduced levels of circulating creatine kinase (a marker of muscle damage), increased range-of-motion recovery, and enhanced strength recovery after the repeated eccentric workout (Pettitt et al. 2005; Balnave & Thompson 1993).

Performing two, six, or ten maximal eccentric contractions has been shown to provide a protective effect for a subsequent repeated bout of twenty-four to fifty maximal muscular contractions weeks later (McHugh 2003). The mechanism that causes the RBE has not been conclusively determined. However, different theories suggest neural input to the muscle, connective tissue restructuring in the muscle and cellular adaptations (an increase in sarcomeres) as possible explanations (McHugh 2003; McHugh et al. 1999).

DIFFERENCES IN THE RESPONSES OF OLD AND YOUNG PERSONS TO ECCENTRIC TRAINING

Older men are not as susceptible as their younger counterparts to the muscle damage caused by eccentric exercise. Another reason why masters athletes do so well when they participate in the Changing Lives Program. There is a stigma against older people, and the impression is that they will take longer to recover after resistance and strength training. This is a false notion, as it depends on the client's program and exercise selection that a professional uses that determines DOMS and other metabolic changes.

Lavender and Nosaka (2006) investigated the responses of older (average age: seventy) and younger (average age: nineteen) males to six sets of five eccentric-exercise reps (at 40% of one-repetition maximum, or 1-RM) targeting the elbow flexors. The younger men experienced more DOMS and showed higher metabolic markers of DOMS (i.e. increased levels of creatine kinase) after the eccentric training. The authors proposed that slight decreases in range of motion (due to age-related changes in muscles) might partially explain the lower levels of DOMS in the older group. In addition, with aging there is a propensity for loss or atrophy (decrease in size) of fast-twitch muscle fibers, which are particularly challenged (leading to DOMS) in eccentric training (Lavender & Nosaka 2006).

Lavender and Nosaka hypothesize that the older adults may instinctively have developed neural inhibitory mechanisms to avoid exercise-induced muscle damage. With females, Ploutz-Snyder et al. (2001) found no difference in DOMS between older women (sixty-six years) and younger women (twenty-three years) in either concentric or eccentric strength training in a twelve-week study evaluating knee extension strength (Jackson, Bubbico, & Kravitz, 2010).

ENTRY-LEVEL CLIENTS: SUBMAXIMAL VS. MAXIMAL ECCENTRIC EXERCISE

As discussed previously, eccentric loading leads to DOMS, especially if the loading occurs in an unaccustomed condition and/or at maximal or near-maximal intensities. During traditional resistance training workouts, the loads of the lifts are typically submaximal (i.e. some percentage of 1-RM). To compare the DOMS effects following maximal versus submaximal eccentric training, Nosaka and Newton (2002) measured muscle damage (of the elbow flexors) in untrained males after completing maximal eccentric exercise bouts (3 sets of 10 repetitions at 100% of 1-RM) with one arm and submaximal eccentric exercise bouts (3 sets of 10 repetitions at 50% 1-RM) with the other arm, 4 weeks apart (Jackson, Bubbico, & Kravitz, 2010).

Findings indicated that in untrained subjects performing eccentric exercise, muscle damage was significantly less and muscles recovered significantly faster after submaximal (50%) loading than after maximal loading. This is meaningful to personal trainers because it shows that too much intensity can cause greater DOMS, which may lead to a drop-off in exercise adherence among these clients.

ECCENTRIC EXERCISE AND 1 RM STRENGTH

Power and strength goals by masters athletes (involved in strength/power sports) are usually determined by one repetition maximum (1 RM). Strength and power athletes extensively focus on 1 RM as a way to gauge and measure strength increases and decreases. An elevated 1 RM allows an exerciser to have a higher relative submaximal training volume – and allows the potential to improve submaximal muscle performance. In a study conducted by Doan et al. (2002), researchers found that 1 RM could be acutely increased by applying a supramaximal load (i.e. 105% of 1-RM) on the eccentric phase of the lift. This acute increase (5% greater than 1-RM) in eccentric loading improved 1 RM concentric performance by five to fifteen pounds for all subjects (Jackson, Bubbico, & Kravitz, 2010).

Theories for why strength increases following eccentric loading include: enhanced neural stimulation to and within muscle, higher stored elastic energy in muscle, and increases in muscle hypertrophy. Neural stimulation within muscle from eccentric exercise causes a greater muscle spindle stretch. The muscle spindle is a stretch receptor in muscle that lies parallel to the contractile proteins (actin and myosin). It is responsive to stretch and speed of stretch. A greater stretch of the muscle spindles activates an increase in firing motor nerves to the muscle, potentially boosting the concentric force of contraction in the muscle fibers (Dietz, Schmidtbleicher & Noth 1979).

Doan and colleagues suggest that supramaximal eccentric training is an excellent tool to have athletes and clients complete in order to break through training plateaus. Hortobágyi et al. (1996) note that in a twelve-week study of isokinetic concentric versus isokinetic eccentric training, subjects experienced more fatigue with the concentric training regimen. The authors conclude that these findings advocate the importance of integrating eccentric training into recreational settings. This further evidence and research solidifies the importance of eccentric programming as an integral method used in the Changing Lives Program.

ECCENTRIC EXERCISE AND REHABILITATION

Rehabilitation programming for masters athletes and other older adults is imperative in the Changing Lives Program. Anterior cruciate ligament reconstruction (ACL-R) rehabilitation continues to be a challenging area of research. Safe and effective methods are constantly being researched. Careful, progressive overloading of the muscle early after surgery is essential to an effective recovery (Jackson, Bubbico, & Kravitz, 2010).

Gerber and colleagues (2009) found that patients performing a twelve-week eccentric training program (along with functional rehabilitation exercises) beginning three weeks after surgery showed greater improvements in quadriceps femoris and gluteus maximus muscle volume and overall function than patients performing a standard rehabilitation protocol of weight-bearing exercise, resistance exercise, and functional training. At a one-year follow-up, the eccentric exercise group had a 50% greater improvement in quadriceps femoris and gluteus maximus muscle volume. Improvement in overall function was significantly greater in this group than in the standard rehabilitation control group (Jackson, Bubbico, & Kravitz, 2010).

Another common injury (especially in athletes) treated in rehabilitation settings is patellar tendinopathy (jumper's knee). Jumper's knee occurs frequently in high-level volleyball, basketball, and soccer players. Using a twelve-week eccentric rehabilitation intervention, Bahr et al. (2006) found no measurable differences between a surgical intervention and eccentric exercise rehabilitation for jumper's knee in a combined athlete and non-athlete group of predominantly men.

With the prevalence of fitness enthusiasts pushing themselves to compete in recreational sports, it is helpful for personal trainers to realize that eccentric training is a viable intervention to use with clients needing post-rehabilitation conditioning. Eccentric exercise methodology is imperative in the development of masters athletes, especially participants in the Changing Lives Program.

ECCENTRIC EXERCISE AND BOOSTING METABOLISM

When most people talk about boosting energy expenditure in exercise, they talk about popular interval training workouts. Now we are raising awareness and educating the fitness community about the eccentric emphasis that should be implemented in programs to have an overall maximized result for burning more calories. The Changing Lives Program harnesses this logic with an all-around purpose to support a multi-faceted approach and give a masters athlete client optimum result and service.

One of the major complaints from adults is they "have no metabolism" or their "metabolism is too slow" or even better, they've "had a slow metabolism all my life." These statements are profoundly not true if one implements proper methods of training and coaching to break physiological barriers to influence superficial and functional changes. The Changing Lives Program has a mission to raise awareness and is responsible for the maximum development for participating clients to improve their metabolism.

Research has found that doing exercise with an eccentric emphasis can raise the resting energy expenditure (REE) of both trained and untrained individuals after a total-body multiset workout (Hackney, Engels & Gretebeck 2008). Hackney and colleagues found that performing a full-body workout with an eccentric emphasis (one-second concentric and three-second eccentric on all exercises) elevated REE approximately 9% after the workout. The REE from resistance exercise is likely caused by recovery and repair factors associated with DOMS, the overall muscle repair process and the energy costs associated with protein synthesis (Hackney, Engels & Gretebeck 2008).

Moreover, eccentric muscle exercises provide many unique features of conditioning benefits. The challenge to fitness professionals is to recognize the potential of this power-generating training method and to structure effective workouts that will benefit clients.

FIFTEEN KEY DISCOVERIES REGARDING ECCENTRIC TRAINING PRINCIPLES

1. Eccentric exercise creates greater force during the eccentric bout, owing to the decreased rate of actin-myosin cross-bridge detachments (Herzog et al. 2008). Clients are therefore capable of working with greater weight during an eccentric exercise.

2. Eccentric contractions use less energy, even though they create more force than concentric actions. This is because during a concentric muscle action one molecule of ATP is used to detach each actin-myosin cross-bridge. However, during an eccentric action some cross-bridges are forcibly detached as a result of the stretching of the muscle fiber, thus using less ATP (McHugh et al. 1999).

3. Some clients feel more muscle "tenderness," as opposed to muscle soreness, from DOMS (Proske & Allen 2005).

4. The only scientific method of using eccentric exercise with clients to markedly reduce DOMS is the repeated bout effect. Completing a bout of eccentric exercises and then repeating the workout one week (or more) later will result in less DOMS after the second workout (Pettitt et al. 2005).

5. For injured clients, eccentric exercise of the "healthy" limb is a viable cross-training option for the immobilized limb (Housh et al. 1998).

6. Older clients are less susceptible to muscle injury from eccentric exercise than their younger counterparts, owing to several inhibiting and physiological

mechanisms (Lavender & Nosaka 2006). Thus, eccentric training is an efficacious strategy to use with older clients.

7. Near-maximal or maximal eccentric muscular contractions should be avoided with "entry-level" clients (Nosaka & Newton 2002). Submaximal loads have been shown to produce much less DOMS and thus may also improve exercise compliance.

8. Resistance exercise programs should include periods of eccentric exercise, as this type of training will provide protection from injury or re-injury (Proske & Allen 2005).

9. For optimal development of muscle strength and size, programs should include both concentric and eccentric training (Proske & Allen 2005).

10. An enhanced submaximal training volume is possible if supramaximal eccentric loading is integrated into the resistance training program (Doan et al. 2002). Supramaximal eccentric training is an excellent tool for athletes and clients who wish to break through training plateaus (Doan et al. 2002).

11. Eccentric training has proven to be a successful post-rehabilitation intervention for lower-body injuries (Bahr et al. 2006).

12. In some research, subjects report less fatigue from eccentric training than from concentric training. These findings support the importance of integrating eccentric training into personal training settings (Hortobágyi et al. 1996).

13. Total-body eccentric emphasis training (i.e. one second-concentric and three- to four-second eccentric contractions) can elevate resting metabolic

rate about 9% (greatest magnitude in first two hours) (Hackney, Engels & Gretebeck 2008).

14. The energy cost of eccentric training is very low, while the magnitude of the force produced is unusually high. Therefore, muscles respond to eccentric training with meaningful changes in strength, size, and power (Lindstedt, LaStayo & Reich 2001).

IS THERE A SUPERIOR METHOD IN PERFORMING ECCENTRIC TRAINING EXERCISES?

Various eccentric training techniques have surfaced in this review, however there are many other eccentric training techniques. With all eccentric training workouts, make sure the client completes an appropriate total body tissue warming (such as low to moderate aerobic exercise for five to ten minutes), followed by appropriate muscle-joint preparation for the ensuing workout. Prior to completing any eccentric exercise, do one traditional warm-up set of the exercise (i.e. concentric followed by eccentric phases) at about 50% of what the client normally lifts.

Below are two eccentric training variations that can be employed with almost all resistance training exercises (Jackson, Bubbico, & Kravitz, 2010).

Eccentric Emphasis Training

- Always begin a client with a light set before beginning any eccentric training. Usually 40-50% of one RM is sufficient to achieve maximum safety, tissue warming, and proper neuromuscular facilitation. Another option is to start with the weight the client normally uses for the particular muscular fitness goal.
- Advise the client do the concentric contraction, lifting the load in a one-second "up."

- Advise clients to perform the eccentric contraction, lowering the load in four to five seconds (thus emphasizing the eccentric phase of the exercise).
- Advise the client to complete eight to ten repetitions (as an example). You will probably need to aid with the concentric lifts as the client starts to fatigue.
- Progress with increased time during the lowering, eccentric emphasis phase.
- Individualize the number of sets based on the client's goals and needs.

Supramaximal Eccentric Training

- Commence with the weight the client normally uses for the particular muscular fitness goal. In this case, let's say the client normally does a ten RM with 100 pounds, meaning ten repetitions with 100 pounds is possible – but an eleventh repetition is not.
- With the supramaximal technique, start with 105% of what the client lifts – in this example, 105 pounds.
- Advise the client to lift the weight in one to two seconds and lower the load in four to five seconds, still emphasizing the eccentric phase of the lift.
- Progressively increase the supramaximal load (for example, 107%, 110%, 115%, up to 125%) as the client appears ready for greater eccentric training challenges.
- Individualize the number of sets according to the client's goals and needs.

Front Squat Eccentric Performance Tip: Be sure the back stays in an upright and in "tight" engagement – do not allow the client to "curl" up or "round" the back. Make sure the knees are in line with the heels to emphasize more glute, hamstring, and posterior fast twitch muscle recruitment. Have the client lower the barbell until the elbows almost touch the quadriceps.

Incline Leg Press Eccentric Performance Tip: Be sure the back stays in full contact with the equipment base – do not allow the client to "curl" up. Make sure the knees are in line with the toes. Have the client lower the platform until the knees almost touch the chest.

Leg Extension Eccentric Performance Tip: Several studies indicate that single-joint exercises are excellent choices for eccentric exercise training because they emphasize specific muscles. To avoid knee stress with this exercise, ensure that the client does not go past a ninety-degree angle on the eccentric phase.

Barbell Curl Eccentric Performance Tip: As with all single-joint exercises, make sure the client does not over-extend the joint at the end of the eccentric phase.

Overhead Press or Bench Press Eccentric Performance Tip: Some clients will start "noodling or wobbling" slightly with the load. In bench press applications, have the client push against the floor with the feet and keep the upper back arched with scapular retraction on the bench for stability. In standing with the barbell, make sure the client performs a pelvic tilt and tucks the tailbone downward to emphasize more glute engagement, core muscle recruitment, and trunk area stability. Also, tell the client to press the barbell "behind them" and push themselves mentally under the barbell as if the barbell was going behind them. This allows the load to align with the spine and optimize results, strength, and stability. Tell the client to focus on lowering the bar straight down in overhead and bench press movements. I have used this technique personally in powerlifting competitions as well in my personal strength programs, and it has yielded tremendous results.

PLYOMETRIC AND SPEED TRAINING APPLICATIONS

One of the best activities to initiate neuromuscular facilitation is the old-fashioned box jump. Box jumps and other plyometric exercises are awesome movements to develop power, strength, and athletic coordination in the lower body and core musculature. Impact exercises help to create bone density and elevate cardiovascular health. Plyometrics is defined as exercise with continual rapid stretching and muscle contraction (as by rebounding and jumping) to gain muscular power.

The Competitive Box Jump Organization (CBJO) was founded in 2012 to develop a competitive sport cultivated from popular jumping exercises. CBJO provides amateur athletes the possibility to compete in an organized activity, and helps with education and safe training methods.

Science-based evidence also proves box jumping and plyometrics are imperative in the development of explosive strength and ability for the masters athlete. In 1996, Holcomb's study titled "The Effectiveness of a Modified Plyometric Program on Power and the Vertical Jump," discovered how people became more powerful when they perform resistance training and plyometrics.

The Changing Lives Program acknowledges these powerful exercises with proper assessment, application, and modification for the benefit of the masters athlete.

Training and developing speed in an athlete's program is essential to the development of a masters athlete. The Changing Lives Program understands this notion very well and is keen on the research, development, and methods used to implement speed in a client's program. Increasing power helps to increase sprinting speed. Masters athletes who play softball, tennis, racquetball, flag football, basketball, as well as those who downhill ski or participate in cross country sports can benefit from increasing speed. Power is defined by the end product of force multiplied by velocity. To simplify these terms, strength is the amount of force we produce, therefore the more force production, the stronger you become. Speed is how fast we produce force. In other words, the faster the rate of production, the greater the speed for the masters athlete.

According to the author of *The Speed Encyclopedia* – and my good friend and colleague – Travis Hansen, "maximizing your strength and speed will always yield the highest output of power and athletic ability, period. The bottom line is if you want phenomenal power and explosiveness, then you have to be able to generate the highest amount of strength in the shortest period of time." The Changing Lives Program uses a multitude of modalities to reproduce variances and options for participants, such as heavy applications of resistance training, kettlebells, barbell or weight lifting, body-weight, and other forms of calisthenics. Whatever application of weight training or body-weight or lighter loads of training, a masters athlete has to develop strength as fast as possible.

Here is a Force-Velocity curve supplied by EliteFTS and published by Jamie Bain:

The force-velocity curve has an x and y axis. The y axis is the horizontal axis that denotes velocity, and the x axis is the vertical axis that denotes force. The curve itself is hyperbolic and shows an inverse relationship between force and velocity (for instance the heavier the weight you lift (force), the slower you lift it (velocity); and vice versa. So various types of training come about on different parts of the force-velocity curve (figure 1). As you go from high force, low velocity to low force, high velocity, you go from max strength work to strength-speed to power to speed-strength to speed (Bain, 2012).

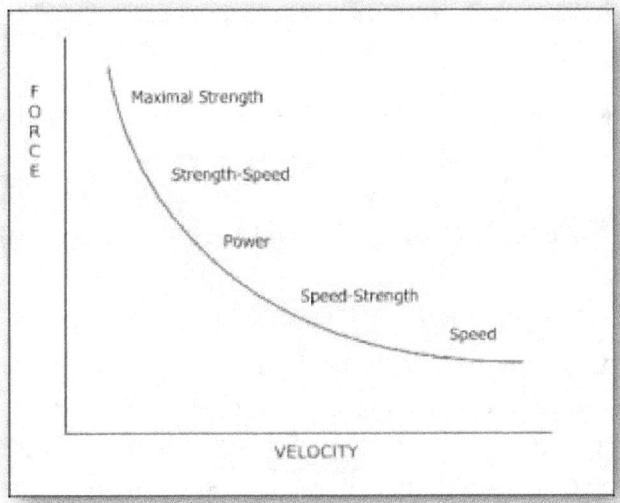

(Figure 1, courtesy of articles.elitefts.com)

So how does this help masters athletes? A desired effect of training is to shift the force-velocity curve to the right (Zatsiorsky 2006) because in sport, speed kills. Training adaptations are specific in nature. Figure 2 shows what happens to the force velocity-curve after strength training (blue) and speed training (green). In advanced athletes, if you train at one end of the force velocity curve, you will improve that part of the curve, but the other will drop-off (Bain, 2012).

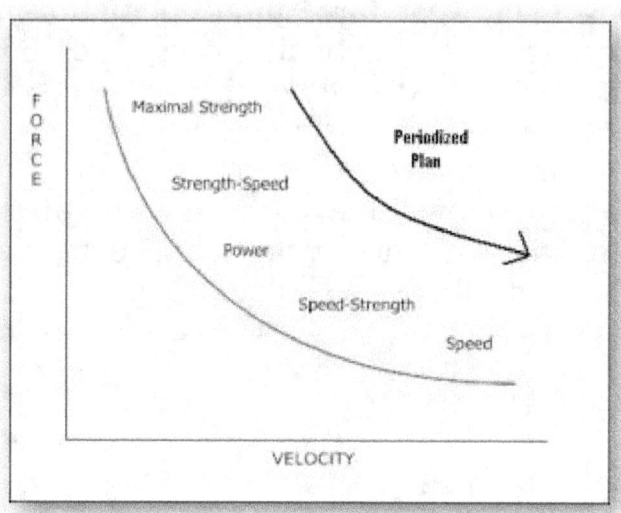

(Figure 2, courtesy of articles.elitefts.com)

The optimal balance is to train the entire force-velocity curve. However how long the athlete spends on training will be depicted by a few variables. Beginners need more time improving maximum strength when compared to experienced athletes. A beginner can also improve speed with developments in maximum strength. As a masters athlete begins a program, he or she will have to emphasize higher velocity speed training, and still work on improving maximum strength, to elevate power capabilities.

Other variables also include the sports that also require different speed and strength characteristics. For example, a lacrosse player will require more strength than a tennis player, however this does not mean the tennis player ignores the strength aspect of the Program. A golf player might require more flexibility drills than a motor-sports racer. Another factor is the position of the athlete in a sport, for instance in softball a pitcher is going to require less speed training compared to a center fielder or leadoff hitter in the lineup. The key to a strength and conditioning expert and qualified fitness professional is to recognize these demands of the masters athlete and adjust the Changing Lives Program specifically, tailoring to individualized needs.

Masters athletes need to train all year and have different training principles applied throughout the season. Max strength should be implemented in the beginning stages of programming, and as the season progresses, emphasis should be placed on speed. A masters athlete does not perform the same max strength block several times at the start of each phase. A client may spend less time on max strength or just execute a more advanced version every time.

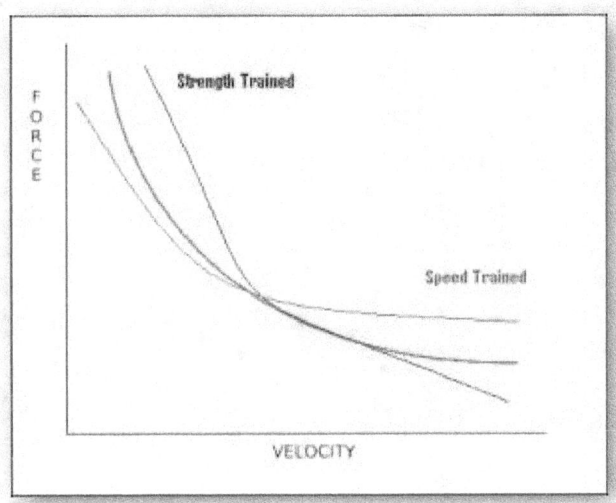

(Figure 3, courtesy of articles.elitefts.com)

How long a masters athlete spends on each stage depends on season, sport, their position in the sport, age, and experience.

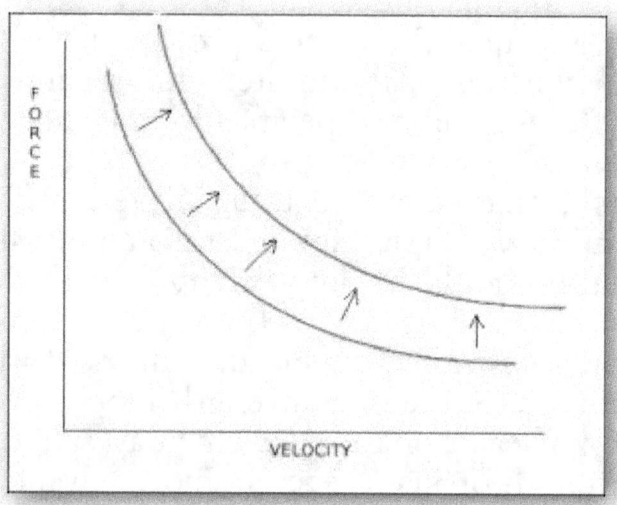

(Figure 4, courtesy of articles.elitefts.com)

VIII

SUCCESSFUL MODELS FOR FITNESS
PROFESSIONALS AND BUSINESS OWNERS

IDEA Health & Fitness Association is the leading re-source for fitness and wellness professionals. In an article on IDEA's website, Valerie Applebaum, MPH, CHES, a certified health education specialist with a master's degree in public health from the University of South Carolina, discusses how "we are in a feeble economy, characterized by sluggish consumer spending and rising unemployment" (2008). In fact, according to the Kiplinger Business Resource Center, "[t]he United States economy in 2008 should limp along, with little or no growth in some quarters and a lousy feeling to many businesses and consumers" (Idaszak, 2008).

When social-economic conditions create a challenging market, the fitness industry must respond quickly in order to weather the storm and prevent financial problems. The good news is that even without drastically altering the way you run your facility, you can shave off unnecessary costs to make it through tough times. Begin by reviewing your budgets and identifying costs that appear superfluous or redundant. Pay special attention to four key areas: staffing, equipment, online presence, and marketing.

STAFFING

1.   Customer Service and a positive attitude are towering principles depicting the cornerstone of all fitness-related facilities and exclusive personal training studios. Taking care of a customer and having excellent interpersonal relations is paramount for businesses. In an industry linked with face-to-face communication, opportunities for staff to interact with potential clients dictates the initiative to sign up for a membership or purchase personal training. Trainers and other front desk personnel who display a positive attitude, superb communication skills, and an ambitious motive to help clients will most likely achieve their business.

   Companies like Regus are leading the competition because of award-winning customer service platforms. Regus Group Companies is a multinational corporation that provides serviced office accommodation in business centers. Regus is the largest provider of executive suites, office space, virtual offices, conference rooms, etc. (Regus, 2013).

   A company's customer service policy is a reflection of how they do business. A musing of how imperative the company values its clients. The Changing Lives Program harnesses this notion as a crucial concept in the philosophy of taking care of face-to-face clients as well as online members. Quality customer service is a key element in the Changing Lives Program because support in these areas influences clients to use and reuse the services and products associated with the Changing Lives Program. Clients are the consumers of DTR Fitness's service, and the key participants of the Changing Lives Program, thus driving the sales that push our programs and services toward exponential growth.

2. Using a proper balance of proactive and reactive approaches will give clients' their due attention, and allow them to feel their concerns are being comprehended. A proactive approach uses the anticipation of a client's needs and actively reaches out to the customer to address those specific needs. This requires gathering information regarding a Changing Lives Program client's satisfaction level. Being proactive in customer service leads to elevated opportunities to reorder a service. A reactive approach, on the other hand, reacts to the client's needs with active listening skills, and includes proper questions regarding a client's needs. Selling is 70-80% listening and 20-30% talking. Implementing this key fundamental approach with staff will transcend efforts to establishing superb rapport with clients.

3. Another effective tool during challenging economic times is to cross-train employees. If employees can handle more than one job, you can combine positions or avoid hiring temporary help during peak periods. Hiring more ambitious and passionate students who are driven and innovative needs to be considered a priority. Interns can do some of the front desk or administrative work, but need to be high energy, and very passionate in customer service and the related field. Looking to local high school or college for students pursuing careers in the fitness industry can be helpful. Passionate and driven students will be thrilled with the work experience, and you will save on

your staffing budget. Passive personality types and less action-oriented individuals will not be considered for employment.

4. Rather than setting a fixed salary, implement incentive pay for employees (Winters, 2000). Providing a base salary approximately 80–85% of overall compensation, with the remaining compensation being tied to performance, motivates staff to become involved in the success of the business.

5. Finally, staff should be trained to take accurate anthropometric measurements when gathering data on the changing physiology of a client. Methods such as skin-fold caliper testing, Bod Pod, Dexascan or bioelectrical impedance (just to name a few) can truly glorify the personalized experience with a client in the Changing Lives Program. Based on scientific research and evidence, error rates when using such anthropometry methods range from 7% to 13%. The key significant concept is retrieving baseline data to determine a line of progression. At the end of the day, numbers are numbers, and using a proven system that has worked throughout our scientific history should be implemented as such to maintain credible and sustainable data collection and service.

EQUIPMENT

Exercise equipment ranks high on the list of health club costs. Fortunately, there are ways you can save significantly on equipment. Making all of your purchases from one company can lower your overall price tag, and many manufacturers offer competitive commercial lease programs that will considerably lower your monthly costs. One of the major benefits of the Changing Lives Program is the lack of bulky machinery and the addition of unconventional cost-saving and unorthodox fitness equipment that saves space. For instance, our program uses TRX suspension training, kettlebells, sandbags, calisthenics, yoga, mat Pilates, stability balls, jump ropes, pull-up and dip bars, jumping platforms and resistance bands, etc.

Another option is to purchase used, demo, refurbished, or re-manufactured equipment for our Olympic weight-lifting applications. Although some dealers use these terms interchangeably, there are key differences. Used equipment is sold "as is" with no guarantees that it will function properly. Demo models were likely not used very often. Refurbished equipment has been cleaned up, inspected, and tested. It works, but there may not be a warranty or return policy. And re-manufactured equipment has been completely dismantled and rebuilt to factory specifications. The paint has been sanded off and reapplied. The gears, cables, bearings, upholstery and electronics have been replaced.

There is no piece of equipment that must be purchased new, as long as you can buy it used through a reputable dealer. Employ research, and ensure that the company you select has after-sale liability insurance in case of possible mishaps with the equipment (due to poor product re-manufacturing). A respectable company will also offer a warranty on all parts and labor. Six months on parts and labor is the industry standard (Eason, 2007).

ONLINE PRESENCE AND MARKETING

1. Choose a website company that can provide you with ample web space, especially if your site is rich

in graphics or has video clips. Your website provider should also offer FTP (File Transfer Protocol) access. FTP allows you to modify your website using your choice of software and quickly upload the changes. This ensures that you can expand your site at any time as your business grows, or if you decide to enhance your online business capabilities. Even when your budget is tight, you need to keep promoting your facility.

2. At first you may believe that big funds are a necessity for marketing and advertising, but you can employ many creative strategies to promote a club on a small budget. Social media is the future of marketing and advertising, and as such it is a great tool that should not be underestimated. Twitter, Facebook, LinkedIn, Google, and YouTube have been monumental in the process of DTR Fitness, LLC. The numerous groups and organizations present in social media have aided our goals of raising awareness and changing lives.

    Develop relationships with owners of local businesses that serve the same target market as you do, such as sporting goods stores, sports injury clinics, and spas. You can partner with these organizations by displaying your marketing materials at their locations, and in exchange letting them display their materials at your gym (Metcalf 2004). Another idea is to swap ad space in your newsletters. Joining the local chamber of commerce can help you network with local businesses to start building these relationships.

3. Help yourself by helping others and being involved in the community. "[S]upport or create a local race

or fun walk," suggests Andrea Metcalf, creator and host of *Fit Today* and owner of MBC Fitness in Westmont, Illinois, who organizes an annual 5K race that starts outside her club on the Saturday after Thanksgiving. "The relationships with the community, chamber and local stores build upon each other."

It is a well-known fact that schools and community centers are cutting back on physical education classes. Use this information to your advantage by volunteering your staff to teach exercise classes at local schools or community centers. Arrange field trips in which students come to the gym to work out and learn about careers in fitness. This act raises your profile in the community and introduces your club to parents and teachers, who are potential members (Mullich 2003).

4. One of the most crucial ways to save on advertising is to ensure that you are using the right media. You can spend thousands of dollars on ads that are simply not targeting true prospective members. Rather than spend a significant portion of your budget on large television ads or national consumer magazine spreads, focus on targeted media in your community such as local lifestyle publications, local cable talk shows, or inserts in newspapers in your geographic area (Mullich, 2003). You will not only reach more potential members but also save money.

Examining your club's expenses may take some time, but the benefits of decreasing spending in challenging economic times are crucial to the survival of the business. You will be amazed at how some little cost cuts here and there add up to major savings for your facility, keeping your budget strong.

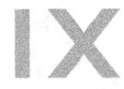

Financial Management

Additional Notes for Fitness Professionals and Coaches

The Changing Lives Program is a value-added service to a public or private health club or fitness studio. It is also a separate service offered to potential customers to take advantage of an incredible life-changing experience. Personal training, semi-private instruction, and other fitness needs will be priced as follows:

Enrollment into the Changing Lives Program requires a minimum of a three-month commitment, and a maximum of one year of continued service. The program will be set up similarly to a gym membership with electronic funds transfer, and members will be billed a monthly premium of $550-$1200 per individual, depending on discounts, or promotions and the number of training sessions serviced. For instance, a member who signs up for a maximum three sessions per week in the Changing Lives Program will incur a monthly $960 fee. Two sessions a week will incur a $500 fee. A health club member who is interested in three sessions a week, nutritional recommendations, phone support, and wellness coaching will incur the $1200 monthly fee.

Monthly fees are set in stone, which includes no sliding fee scale. Clients will be charged monthly with payments up front. The drop-in rate for sessions three times a week or more average $85 per meeting, and less than three times a week $95 per sitting. Youths, adults, elders, and disabled persons will be accommodated with similar fee schedules. The Changing Lives Program will use the latest fitness trends and tools to create maximum physical, mental, and spiritual well-being.

BUDGET

The Changing Lives Program began as a grassroots organization mainly because of a lack of resources available. An ideal circumstance for the Changing Lives Program is an investor or investors who have a strong interest in our mission and can assist acquiring a large facility, such as one ranging from 30,000 to 100,000 square feet with multiple floors. In the short term, DTR Fitness is working together with the Changing Lives Program to start a small facility of approximately 1,300 square feet of space in a commercial property located in South Reno, Nevada. The rent or lease of the property is approximately fifty-five cents per square foot, plus utilities, insurance, liability, and other city and building permits.

Equipment needed for the facility to provide DTR Fitness, LLC and the Changing Lives Program's services is approximately $20,000. (An attached document of budget for equipment and other necessary items for facility can be provided with more detailed explanation.) Functional equipment such as TRX suspension trainers, Kettlebells, Medicine balls, and resistance bands will alleviate high end cost for expensive equipment that normal public facilities such as 24 Hour Fitness and Fitness Connection have to deal with. The other costs of proper gym flooring (two to three dollars per square foot), additional paint, and other materials needed for renovations or maintenance also necessitate consideration. Advertising and marketing will be budgeted to just $500 to $8,000 per month, depending on resources and availability. Other costs involve merchandise – a budget of $500 per month on clothing inventory to produce a small (10-15%) profit margin to assist in marketing and advertising promotions for the program and exposure for the facility.

Staff will include two qualified fitness professionals with duties involving customer service, logistics, building maintenance and upkeep, constant monitoring and evaluation of participating members, personal training, group class instruction, and nutritional guidance. Budget for staff will be a fixed salary of $2,000 per month to start. Once business accelerates and shows growth, expansion will increase revenue sharing, profits, and possible relocation or expansion to a larger facility.

X

New Possibilities

Masters athletes participating in this program can accomplish a multitude of goals. One might become a fashion model. Another might be an aspiring athlete in a competitive sport. Some masters athletes simply have the goal to be more physically fit – to climb Mount Everest or partake in a triathlon. The opportunities for the Changing Lives Program are limitless. Believing in the system and comprehending the program will give masters athletes new goals, push them to new heights, and allow them to overcome challenges that they may have struggled with during previous exercise programs. This is a major breakthrough in the evolution of exercise science and human kinetics for the development and potential for a masters athlete.

Progressing a client from walking two to three miles per day several times during a month to running a marathon is a major accomplishment, and requires a multifaceted approach to exercise programming and protocol. Mistakes people often make is trying to implement the end-all-be-all approach with training methodology. There is no single method that can create success. Success requires a multitude of proven research and result-based evidence to give clients what they want and truly deserve.

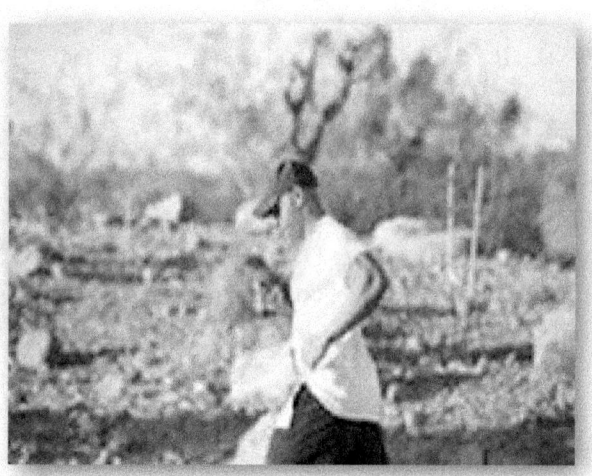

Dietrich training for a half marathon
in 2008.

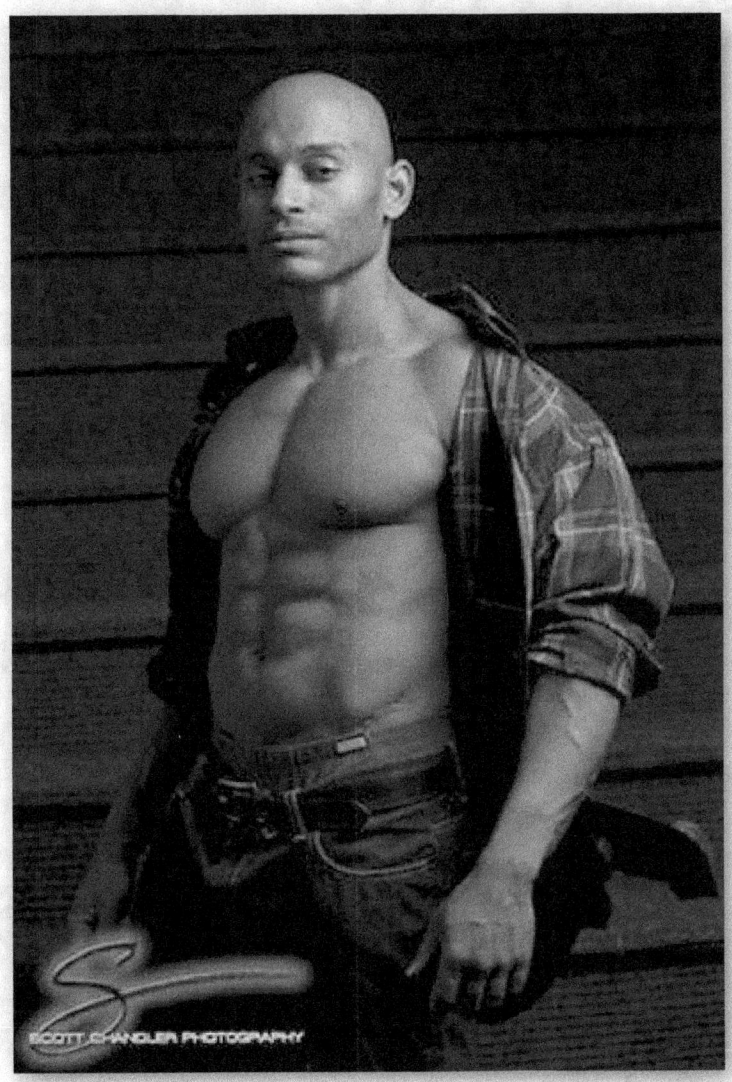

Dietrich modeling photo

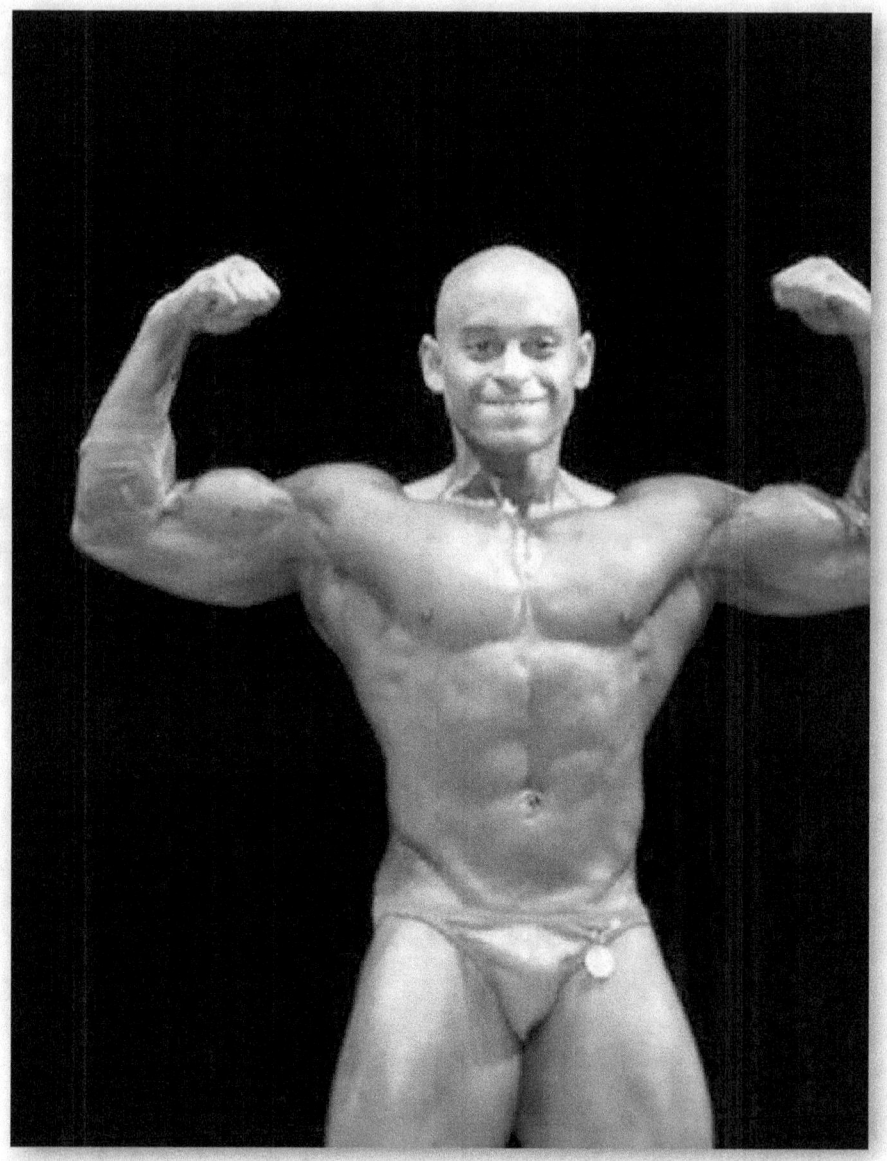

Dietrich Tahoe Show Bodybuilding competition 2011

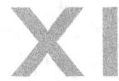

XI

Conclusion

In retrospect, if the goal is to improve physical capacity or to compete at a higher level, people who are active, mature adults are compelled to state that exercise is the only concept that keeps them healthy, strong, and feeling like they're twenty.

I wrote *50 Fit Shades of Fitness* to revolutionize the way mature adults approach fitness by increasing awareness and removing mental blocks to accomplish new active goals and promote long-term physical changes.

Seven years of research and eighteen years of experience went into this book to help people comprehend on a higher level the realms of possibilities of achieving fitness goals and reversing the aging process. Why settle for less? Why do the same things that other people do? Why not attempt to change your life and be more functional, increase vitality, feel better, look great naked at forty-five or fifty-four years of age, have a family and work a full schedule and still look and feel like you're twenty-five years old? These are questions people have to ask themselves in order to achieve a new comprehension of long-term sustainability in health and fitness. All things are possible for masters athletes! Older adults need to realize the potential of what can be accomplished with a sound physical fitness program and great coaching implementation.

Our exciting new fitness program is developed to change people's lives every single day. We discussed the mission, purpose, business philosophy, key elements, best practices, and financial management aspect of the program. Adults over thirty-five can accomplish their goals if they set forth with hard work, dedication, commitment, and knowledge of the mission at hand. All masters athletes, regardless of shape, size, sports background, and gender can all experience immediate extraordinary changes in their lifestyle. The goal of this program is to implement resistance training, cardiovascular exercise, flexibility, nutrition, and mental coaching into a life-changing experience for all participants. The Changing Lives Program uses the latest fitness trends and tools to create maximum physical, mental, and spiritual well-being, and empower participants to have more confidence in their ability to maintain lifelong adherence to health and wellness. The purpose is always changing lives.

As a masters athlete myself, I believe that there should be fun and functional programs created to enhance the development of older adults. I've grown tired of the misconception that age is an excuse for not being able to physically perform an exercise program. Those days are gone, and with the Changing Lives Program, masters athletes will have a unique and unconventional approach to developing their physical capabilities and achieving their goals.

2015 and beyond will embark a new era of innovation and creativity. The present and future era will advance and we will discover what was once considered physically impossible. The Changing Lives Program will continue to evolve and teach masters athletes how to surpass any limitation. From rock-climbing to ultra-marathons, Olympic lifting to tough mudder, and skiing to team sports, the

Changing Lives Program will be available to help you reach your desired results. Imagine fitness regimens for masters athletes which consist of unconventional body weight exercises, and exercise tools which focus on multi-joint motion, creativity, and functional movement patterns. Envision a program which helps an array of individuals, from thirty-five-year-olds to elders. Well, the Changing Lives Program is here to do just that, and will redefine how we view exercise and results for active adults.

Now, let's get into the best shape of our lives.

References

Applebaum, V. MPH (2008). IDEA Health & Fitness Association. Best practices: staying strong in a weak economy. Retrieved Nov. 21, 2008, from Idea Fitness Manager, Volume 5, No. 3, July 2008.

Baechle, T., & Earle, R. (2008). *Essentials of Strength and Conditioning* (3rd ed.). Champaign, IL: Human Kinetics.

Bain, J. (2012). The Force-Velocity Curve. Information retrieved March 12, 2013 from http://articles. elitefts.com/training-articles/sports-training/ the-force-velocity-curve/

Bahr, R, Bjorn, F., Sverre, L., and Engebretsen, L. (2006). Surgical treatment compared with eccentric training for patellar tendinopathy (Jumper's knee). Journal of Bone and Joint Surgery, 88 (8) 1689-1698.

Baker, J., et al. (2006). Effects of age on testosterone responses to resistance exercise and musculoskeletal variables in men. *Journal of Strength and Conditioning Research*, 20 (4), 874-81.

Balnave, C.D., and Allen, D.G. (1995). Intracellular calcium and force in single mouse muscle fibres following repeated contractions with stretch. Journal of Physiology, 488: 25-36.

Balnave, C.D., and Thompson, M.W. (1993). Effect of training on eccentric exercise-induced muscle damage. Journal of Applied Physiology, 75 (4), 1545-1551.

Brown, S.J., Child, R.B., Day, S.H., and Donnelly, A.E. (1997). Exercise-induced skeletal muscle damage and adaptation following repeated bouts of eccentric muscle contractions. Journal of Sports Science, 15, 215-222.

Bryant, C., & Green, D. (2009). *ACE Advanced Health and Fitness Specialist Manual.* San Diego: ACE.

Bubbico, A. & Kravitz, L. (2010). Eccentric Exercise: A Comprehensive Review of a Distinctive Training Method.

Candow, D.G., et al. (2011). Short-term heavy resistance training eliminates age-related deficits in muscle mass and strength in healthy older males. *Journal of Strength and Conditioning Research*, 25(2), 326-33.

Clark, N. (2012). Personal communication. Retrieved March 28, 2012.

Cummings, K. (Gold's Gym Operations Mgr.), personal communication. Retrieved October 10, 2008.

Dejean, D. (2000-2010). Retrieved April 1, 2010 from http://dtrfitness.net/index.html

Dietz, V., Schmidtbleicher, D. and Noth. J. (1979). Neuronal mechanisms of human locomotion. Journal of Neurophysiology. 42(5), 1212-1222.

Doan, B.K., Newton, R.U., Marsit, J.L., Triplett-McBride, N., Koziris, L.P., Fry, A.C., and Kraemer, W.J. (2002). Effects of increased eccentric loading on bench press 1RM. Journal of Strength & Conditioning Research, 16(1), 9-13.

Eason, J. (2007). Buying used. *Fitness Management* (Aug. 2007).

Enoka, R.M. (1996). Eccentric contractions require unique activation strategies by the nervous system. Journal of Applied Physiology, 81: 2339-2346.

Gerber, J.P., Marcus, R.L., Dibble, L.E., Greis, P.E., Burks, R.T., LaStayo, P.C. (2009). Effects of early progressive eccentric exercise on muscle size and function after anterior cruciate ligament reconstruction: A 1-year follow-up study of a randomized clinical trial. Journal of Physical Therapy. 89(1): 52-59.

Gettman, L. R., & Pollock, M. L. (1981). Circuit weight training: A critical review of its physiological benefits. The Physician and Sportsmedicine, 9, 44-60.

Hansen, T. (2013). The Speed Encyclopedia: A team sports athlete's complete guide to speed development.

Harris, C., et al. (2004). The effect of resistance-training intensity on strength-gain response in the older adult. *Journal of Strength and Conditioning Research, 18* (4), 833-38.

Harris, K. A., & Holly, R. G. (1987). Physiological response to circuit weight training in borderline hypertensive subjects. Medicine and Science in Sports and Exercise, 19, 246-252.

Hackney, K.J., Engels, H.J., and Gretebeck, R.J. (2008). Resting energy expenditure and delayed-onset muscle soreness after full-body resistance training with an eccentric concentration. Journal of Strength and Conditioning Research. 22(5): 1602-1609.

Hempel, L. S., & Wells, C. L. (1985). Cardiorespiratory cost of the nautilus express circuit. The Physician and Sportsmedicine, 13, 82-97.

Herzog, W., Leonard, T.R., Joumaa, V. and Mehta, A. (2008). Mysteries of muscle contraction. Journal of Applied Biomechanics, 24, 1-13.

Holcomb, W. R.; Lander, J. E.; Rutland, R. M.; Wilson, G. D. (1996). The Effectiveness of a Modified Plyometric Program on Power and the Vertical Jump.

Housh, D.J., Housh, T.J., Weir, J.P., Weir, L.L., Evetovich, T.K., & Donlin, P.E. (1998). Effects of unilateral eccentric-only dynamic constant external resistance training on quadriceps femoris cross-sectional area. Journal of Strength & Conditioning Research, 12(3), 192-198.

Hortobagyi, T., Zheng, D., Weidner, M., Lambert, N., Westbrook, S., and Houmard, J. (1995). The influence of aging on muscle strength and muscle fiber characteristics with special reference to eccentric strength. Journal of Gerontology, 50, B399-B406.

Hortobagyi, T., Hill, J.P., Houmard, J.A., Fraser, D.D., Lambert, N.J., Israel, R.G. (1996). Adaptive responses to muscle lengthening, and shortening in humans. Journal of Applied Physiology, 80(3), 765-772.

Hurley, B.F., Hanson, E.D., & Sheaff, A.K. (2011). Strength training as a countermeasure to aging muscle and chronic disease. *Sports Medicine, 41*(4), 289-306.

International Health, Racquet and Sports club Association (IHRSA 2008). Through annual surveys, the IHRSA Research Department collects key operational data related to health club industry benchmarks, best practices, and trends. ... Retrieved Nov. 22, 2008, from cms.ihrsa.org/index.cfm?fuseaction=pageview page&pageId=18735 – http://cms.ihrsa.org/index.cfm?fuseaction=Page.viewPage&pageId=18737&nodeID=15

Idaszak, J. (2008). 2008 economy: On the edge of recession. Retrieved Apr. 20, 2008.

Jackson, L.M. (2010). Eccentric Exercise by Aaron Bubbico and Len Kravitz, PhD. Retrieved from IDEA health & Fitness Cec/CEU course.

Kraemer, W.J., Fleck, S.J., & Deschenes, M.R. (2012). *Exercise Physiology: Integrating Theory and Application.* Baltimore: Lippincott, Williams and Wilkins.

Kravitz, L. (2012). ACSM health and fitness conference summit & exposition. Las Vegas, NV. Personal communication retrieved March 27, 2012.

Kravitz, L. (1996). The fitness professional's complete guide to circuits and intervals. *IDEA Today, 14*(1), 32–43.

Lamb, D.G. (2009). Mechanisms of excitation-contraction uncoupling relevant to activity-induced muscle fatigue. Applied Physiology, Nutrition, and Metabolism, 34: 368-372.

Lavender, A.P, & Nosaka, K. (2006). Comparison between old and young men for changes in makers of muscle damage following voluntary eccentric exercise of the elbow flexors. Applied Physiology, Nutrition, and Metabolism. 31, 218-225.

Lewis, J.A., Lewis, M.D., Packard, T. (2007). Management of human service programs. Chapter 11: Leading and Changing Human Service Organizations. 4th ed. Brooks Cole.

Lian, O.B., Engebretsen, L, Bahr, R. (2005). Prevalence of jumper's knee among elite athletes from different sports: a cross-sectional study. American Journal of Sports Med. 33: 561-567.

Lindstedt S.L., LaStayo P.C., and Reich T.E. (2001). When active muscles lengthen: Properties and consequences of eccentric contractions. News Physiological Science. 16, 256-261.

Mathews, D. K., & Fox, E. L. (1976). The physiological basis of physical education and athletics.

Metcalf, A. (2004). Marketing with little or no money. *Fitness Business Pro* (Aug. 1).

McCall, P. (2013). Performance training for masters athletes. *Idea Fitness Journal* (Nov. & Dec. 2013).

McCrory, J.L., et al. (2009). Thigh muscle strength in senior athletes and healthy controls.
Journal of Strength and Conditioning Research, 23(9), 2430-36.

McHugh, M.P. (2003). Recent advances in the understanding of the repeated bout effect: the protective effect against muscle damage from a single bout of eccentric exercise. Scandinavian Journal of Medicine & Science in Sports 2003: 13: 88-97.

McHugh, M.P., Connolly, D.A.J., Easton, R.G., and Gleim, G.W. (1999). Exercise-induced muscle damage and potential mechanisms for the repeated out effect. Sports Medicine, 27(3): 151-170.

Mullich, J. (2003). Advertising on a budget. *Fitness Business Pro* (Apr. 1).

Norvell, N., & Belles, D. (1993). Psychological and physical benefits of circuit weight training in law enforcement personnel. Journal of Consulting and Clinical Psychology, 61, 520-527.

Nosaka, K., Sakamoto, K., Newton, M. and Sacco, P. (2001). How long does the protective effect on eccentric exercise-induced muscle damage last? Medicine & Science in Sport & Exercise, 33, 1490-1495.

Nosaka, K., and Newton, M. (2002). Difference in the magnitude of muscle damage between maximal and submaximal eccentric loading. Journal of Strength and Conditioning Research, 16(2), 202-208.

Parratt, V. (Saint Mary's Health & Fitness Center Fitness Mgr.), personal communication. Retrieved October 21, 2008.

Peterson M, Alvar B, Rhea M (2006). The Contribution of Maximal Force Production to Explosive Movement Among Young Collegiate Athletes. *Journal of Strength and Conditioning Research* 20(4): 867–73.

Pettitt, R. W., Symons, D. J., Eisenman, P.A., Taylor, J. E., White, Andrea, T. (2005). Repetitive eccentric strain at long muscle length evokes the repeated bout effect. Journal of Strength and Conditioning Research, 19(4), 918-924.

Phillips, W. (2004). Staffing and Strategy: The Hidden Calamity in Many Health Clubs. Retrieved Oct. 22, 2008, from http://www.rexonline.org/showbriefs.php?action=sscalamity

Ploutz-Snyder, L.L, Giamis, E.L., Formikell, M., and Rosenbaum, A.E. (2001). Resistance training reduces susceptibility to eccentric-induced muscle dysfunction in older women. Journal of Gerontology, 56A, B384-B390.

Proske, U. and Allen, T.J. (2005). Damage to skeletal muscle from eccentric exercise. Exercise and Sports Science Reviews, 33(2), 98-104.

Regus Group Companies (2013). Retrieved March 2, 2013 from http://www.regus.com/about-us/index.aspx

Robey, H., & Kazob, F. (Owners of Fitness Enterprises), personal communication. Retrieved October 16, 2008.

Sorani, R. (1966). Circuit training. Dubuque, IA: Wm. C. Brown.

Stone, W. J., & Kroll, W. A. (1986). Sports conditioning and weight training (2nd ed). Boston: Allyn and Bacon, Inc.

Winters, C. (2000). Budgeting 101. *Fitness Business Pro* (Nov. 1).

Yacenda, J. (CEO of Dreams Foundation, Inc.), (2010). Personal communication. Retrieved October 21, 2010.

Yeung, E.W. and Allen, D.G. (2004). Stretch activated channels in stretch-induced muscle damage: role in muscular dystrophy. Clinical and Experimental Pharmacology and Physiology. 31:551-556.

Zatsiorsky V, Kraemer J (2006). *Science and Practice of Strength Training*. Champaign, Illinois: Human Kinetics.

Originality Statement

The submitted manuscript is my original work. I have cited and acknowledged all materials, ideas, and words of others that I have used, adapted, or paraphrased in this document.
  Submitted by: Dietrich Dejean

www.ingramcontent.com/pod-product-compliance
Lightning Source LLC
Chambersburg PA
CBHW071208280526
45787CB00002B/604

9 781505 638363